WAR AND THE HEALTH OF NATIONS

WAR AND THE HEALTH OF NATIONS

ZARYAB IQBAL

STANFORD UNIVERSITY PRESS
Stanford, California

Stanford University Press

Stanford, California

Printed in the United States of America on acid-free, archival-quality paper

Library of Congress Cataloging-in-Publication Data

Iqbal, Zaryab.
    War and the health of nations / Zaryab Iqbal.
       p. cm.
    Includes bibliographical references and index.
    ISBN 978-0-8047-5881-9 (cloth : alk. paper)
       1. War—Health aspects. 2. War—Medical aspects. 3. War and society.
    4. Public health. I. Title.
    RA646.I67   2010
    362.1—dc22   2009029235

Typeset by Westchester Book Group in 10/14 Minion

I dedicate this book to my parents

CONTENTS

Appendixes

TABLES AND FIGURES

ACKNOWLEDGMENTS

THE PROCESS OF CRAFTING THIS BOOK has made me recognize the importance of professional and personal support systems in our ability to pursue scholarly work, and how much we benefit from existing academic infrastructures. Since beginning this project, I have accumulated many debts of gratitude; support from numerous individuals and institutions has been invaluable in its completion. This project began as my PhD dissertation at Emory University, where I benefited tremendously from the encouraging and inspiring scholarly environment of the Political Science Department. My adviser, David Davis, provided me with constant support throughout my graduate career and taught me to "think outside the box." His encouragement was instrumental in helping me come up with a unique dissertation topic, which later morphed into this book. Dan Reiter, Suzanne Werner, and Eric Reinhardt offered valuable comments and suggestions, as well as general support and encouragement, for the improvement of the project.

I owe a great deal to the Department of Political Science and its faculty at the University of South Carolina (USC) for providing me with an excellent working environment during the early years of my career. My discussions with Harvey Starr contributed greatly to the development of this project, and I am very grateful to him for the interest that he has taken in my professional growth; I thank him for being a superb mentor, colleague, and friend. I also benefited immensely from my interactions with a number of other colleagues at USC, including Ann Bowman, Roger Coate, David Darmofal, Jill Frank, Don Puchala, Don Songer, and Neal Woods.

I am also very fortunate to be part of the collegial, supportive, and academically rigorous Department of Political Science at Pennsylvania State University. I would like to thank my colleagues at Penn State for motivating me through the final stages of this book project, particularly Donna Bahry, Frank Baumgartner, Scott Bennett, Doug Lemke, and Glenn Palmer. I want to offer special thanks to James Eisenstein for his comments on the manuscript, and I appreciate Julie Pacheco's help in proofreading.

The quality of this book has been significantly enhanced by the comments and suggestions of two anonymous reviewers chosen by Stanford University Press. I also appreciate the assistance that I have received from the editorial staff of the Press, especially Stacy Wagner and Jessica Walsh.

I would like to thank my sisters and parents for their love and support over the years. Finally, I would like to acknowledge Christopher Zorn for the prodigious role he has played in the cultivation of this project, and for keeping me going through the best of times and the worst of times. At each stage of the project, I have gained from his insights and assistance. In addition to his indispensable advice on methodology, he has been a source of unwavering support and encouragement. I thank him for inspiring me as a political scientist, for challenging me to do my best, and for believing in me.

WAR AND THE HEALTH OF NATIONS

1

INTRODUCTION

SINCE THE END OF WORLD WAR II, there have been numerous interstate and intrastate conflicts resulting in millions of deaths and billions of dollars' worth of destruction. Yet scholars have paid very little attention to the consequences of conflict, in particular to its social consequences. The World Health Organization's (WHO) 2002 *World Report on Violence and Health* revealed that 1.6 million people die each year due to violence, including collective violence such as conflicts within or between states, and a large number of the people who lose their lives due to militarized conflict are noncombatants. The 25 largest instances of conflict in the twentieth century led to the deaths of approximately 191 million people, and 60 percent of those fatalities occurred among people who were not engaged in fighting (World Health Organization 2002a). One of the most significant effects of war is the toll it takes on the health and well-being of a population beyond the immediate casualties of combat. In this book, I assess the costs of armed conflict by explaining the relationship between armed conflict and public health.

War leads to direct casualties and deaths during combat; violent conflict also results in widespread death and disability among the civilian populations that are affected either as collateral damage or as deliberate targets. For instance, Russia lost 10.1 percent of its population during World War II,

Korea lost 10 percent of its population during the Korean War, and Vietnam lost 13 percent of its population during the Vietnam War (Garfield and Neugut 1997). In addition to direct deaths and injuries caused by combat among the military and civilian populations, conflict results in conditions that contribute to the spread of disease and retardation of health care systems, such as the influenza outbreak during World War I, which killed more people than combat-related deaths. The disease and disability during and after armed conflict is often accompanied by states' inability to meet the public health needs of their populations if their health care infrastructure has been damaged or destroyed. Moreover, wars are associated with the creation of suboptimal health conditions that result in hazards such as famine, epidemics, weapons-induced pollution, lack of clean water, poor sanitation, and general indigence. Consequently, the population is exposed to new health threats without access to proper health care.

Studying the relationship between conflict and health is particularly important in light of the nature of conflicts in the current international system. Most of the recent and ongoing conflicts in the world are civil or intrastate wars that lead to large-scale devastation of a state's infrastructure since all the fighting occurs on the territory of one state. This amplifies the conditions that deteriorate the health of societies. Civil conflict is also highly likely to result in displacement of people as refugees or internally displaced persons, exposing communities to health menaces. The crisis in Liberia effectively demonstrates the suffering civil war can inflict on a population. In June 2003, as the Liberian capital of Monrovia was engulfed in violence, the city experienced an outbreak of cholera, and within three months, 6,353 cases of cholera had been reported (World Health Organization 2003). The civil war made it impossible for either Liberian authorities or international agencies to carry out the extensive process of water chlorination that could halt further spread of the disease. Moreover, afflicted people were unable to access medical facilities due to the security situation. In September 2003, the WHO reported that only 32 percent of the Liberian population had access to clean water, no more than 30 percent of the population had access to latrines, and there had been no regular garbage collection in Monrovia since 1996. The SKD Stadium, the largest camp for internally displaced people in Monrovia, housed about 45,000 people who "cook and sleep in any sheltered spot they can find, in hallways and in tiny slots under the stadium seats," with six nurses in the health center for 400 daily patients (World Health Organization 2003). After the civil war, the life expectancy in Liberia remains 41 years.

Examples of devastating effects of violent conflict on public health abound in recent decades. In the Sudan, prolonged conflict has exposed the population to diseases such as yellow fever, malnutrition, displacement of large groups, poverty, and famine. The Iraqi society experienced near destruction of their health care system, previously one of the best in the Middle East, during the first Gulf War. Public health in Iraq continued on a path of steady decline for a decade of international sanctions and internal repression, after which the general and health infrastructures were subjected to a second war. In 1993, Iraq's water supply was estimated at 50 percent of prewar levels (Hoskins 1997) and war-related postwar civilian deaths numbered about 100,000 (Garfield and Neugut 1997). In 2006, approximately 2 million people were internally displaced in Iraq (United Nations High Commissioner for Refugees 2007).

For every interstate or civil war, populations of states suffer short-term and long-term effects on their health and well-being. To understand the real cost of violent conflict, it is necessary to take into account the *human* cost of war. Violent conflict can have economic, social, political, and environmental consequences; yet, while a large number of conflict studies focus on causes of conflict, the literature about the consequences of conflict—and in particular the health consequences—remains relatively scarce. While scholars have examined some aspects of the economic and political consequences of conflict, far less work has been done on the manner in which conflict undermines public health. The effects of conflict on a society continue long after the actual fighting has ceased, and understanding the social consequences of war is integral to estimating the true cost of conflict.

The effect of war on population well-being is closely associated with national and global security. The traditional approaches to studying security focus primarily on state-level factors. The idea of security is generally considered synonymous with protecting the territory and national interests of a state from external aggression or unwelcome interference. Once a state is able to safeguard its military, territorial, and political interests from outside threats, it is perceived to have attained national security. Particularly during the Cold War era, realist notions of security dictated that foreign policy and state leaders remain unrelentingly occupied with the pursuit of military superiority. The emphasis of neorealist theory on states as the single most important entity in the international system led to the deprecation of the interests of sub-state actors. Entities without sovereignty did not warrant attention at the international level, and what occurred within the borders of a sovereign state was to be addressed at the domestic level. Only threats to the security and existence of states were considered detrimental to global security and thus worthy of international attention and action.

In stark contrast to this conventional perspective, the emerging notion of *human security* considers first and foremost the security of state populations; this perspective asserts that the factors that engender insecurity among the people living within states are not limited to perpetuation of the state. Instead, the security of people is inextricably bound up with their quality of life and, therefore, threats to their security include a range of social and economic issues beyond the territorial integrity of their states. Elements of human security include economic security, political security, access to food and health care, personal and community security, and environmental security (United Nations Development Programme 1994). The occurrence of violent international conflict can adversely affect any or all of these factors and amplify the insecurity of people in the affected state. However, the absence of militarized conflict does not guarantee the elimination of these threats to human security. In order to gain an adequate understanding of whether people—and not merely states—are secure, the various components of human security must be addressed rather than conflating the security of people with the security of their state. The shift from state security to human security is necessitated by the salience and the global nature of the issues that threaten the security of populations. Problems like environmental degradation and disease proliferation do not just threaten the security of people in a single state; these problems can easily reach global magnitude.

Although the literature on the concept of human security offers varying definitions of what constitutes the security of people, there is a clear agreement that health is an important component of security. Human security entails the ability of people to maintain a quality of life that does not fall below the level at which they feel secure. Adequate provision of public health is important in enabling people to achieve a secure quality of life and to be functional enough to maintain their lifestyle. It is the security of populations, rather than states, that makes the world secure. State security is important in that people cannot be secure if the existence of the states in which they live is threatened. However, students of security must go beyond state security to understand the true nature of human security. Violent conflict is accepted as a major threat to the security of states; it is also a formidable threat to the security of state populations. One way in which conflict decreases the security of people is by causing a decline in provision of public health. Since the health of a population is an integral component of the security of communities and individuals, studying the effect of conflict on health is an important contribution to the understanding of human security. And human security, due to its focus on the well-being of populations, is a better framework within which to assess international security than the traditional approach of viewing the security of states as the best indicator of global security.

Studying the relationship between conflict and public health is valuable for scholars, policy makers, practitioners, and the general population. Understanding this relationship adds to the scholarly literature about the consequences of conflict by focusing attention on its effects on public health. A rigorous social scientific exploration of this topic provides policy makers with relevant information for decisions regarding public health, including but not limited to allocation of resources for health purposes. Moreover, a wider knowledge base on this topic would enable health care workers and public health practitioners to develop a clearer understanding of a significant influence on the health of a society and, therefore, to better perform their duties.

The implications of this project have broad relevance due to the interconnectedness of the issues involved in the relationship between conflict

and health. The ideas of human security have already become an important force in foreign and domestic policy making. Canada, Japan, Norway,
and a number of other states are members of the Human Security Network
and are actively incorporating considerations of human security into their
policy decisions. An understanding of the effect of war on health would
inform the security policies of states as the costs of war become clearer.
Just as the financial cost of waging war is taken into consideration before
embarking on military action, the health cost—if properly understood—
would also be a factor in the decision to go to war. Further, an emphasis
on human security and health is likely to influence budgetary trade-offs
between defense and social spending. In addition to policy makers at the
national level, this study holds relevance for practitioners and international
organizations in the realms of security, development, health, and human
rights. Health care is closely related to broader issues of development and
the effect of conflict on health calls for active participation by humanitarian
agencies. Understanding how conflict affects public health serves two chief
purposes in the policy/practice arena. First, it enables policy makers and
practitioners in national governments and international governmental and
nongovernmental organizations to formulate more effective strategies for
dealing with humanitarian emergencies as well as long-term health issues,
such as disabilities and preventive health care. Second, it illuminates a significant social cost of conflict, making violent conflict less attractive. The
higher the projected cost of violent conflict, the more likely states and groups
are to seek nonviolent means of conflict resolution. Most important, this
study is relevant to the people whose security it addresses. An important
element of human security is the empowerment of people to enhance their
own security. Comprehending the costs of war influences the perception of
war among populations and affects public opinion and decisions regarding
political participation.

The academic audience for this study is also wide and diverse. The examination of the effect of conflict on health draws on, and contributes to, the
fields of conflict processes, development, economics, and public health.
The range of sociopolitical and economic factors involved in assessing the
costs and consequences of war reflects the interconnectedness of various

academic disciplines in social scientific work. Conflict and security scholars maintain a profound interest in the causes and consequences of war; this study examines an important impact of conflict within a broader framework of security than has been employed in previous work. The close relationships among poverty, development, war, economics, and health extend the scope of this project to development economists and public health scholars. Studying the security of people rather than the security of states calls for an integrative approach in scholarship. Issues of military security of states could be delegated to scholars of war, but the broad and complex nature of human security warrants a multidisciplinary approach. Since this study is based in the human security framework and contributes to the understanding of human security, it holds relevance for scholars in any discipline that deals with issues that influence the quality of life of populations.

The impact of violent conflict on public health disrupts the lives of populations in the immediate and short term by causing death and destruction, and in the medium and long term due to the inability of communities to meet their possibly escalated health care needs. War results in large numbers of deaths among combatants as well as the civilian populations and destroys many aspects of community life that are necessary to meet the health care needs of people. The violence and devastation of war results in destruction of important elements of the infrastructure, as well as in diversion of scarce resources from social and health spending to military expenditures. As violence pervades the society, it becomes an accepted means of resolving issues and leads to domestic violence and increased crime (Levy and Sidel 1997). Hence violent conflict has serious and lasting effects on public health, and this book explores questions regarding the way in which these negative effects occur. Conflict adversely affects public health and the exploration of this relationship in this book makes theoretical and conceptual, as well as methodological, contributions to the disciplines of political science and public health. The question of how conflict affects public health holds interest for both scholars and policy makers, and this work is an attempt to offer a social scientific analysis of the issue.

The main argument in this book is that violent conflict has serious direct and indirect effects on the health of a society and that war undermines the well-being of populations through a range of mechanisms. Militarized violence obviously has a negative effect on the well-being of a society due to death and injury; but war also results in indirect effects on health through decreased efficiency of health care systems, prevalent disabilities among the population, and the spread of disease. History reveals that more soldiers lose their lives due to infectious diseases than through direct armed conflict (Foege 1997). In this book, I explore the multiple dimensions of the war and health relationship and analyze the linkages among armed conflict, political and socioeconomic influences, societal capacities, and population well-being. Below I present an overview of the organization of the book.

As mentioned above, this study is motivated by the human security framework. In Chapter 2, I discuss the concept of human security and argue that this perspective offers a more appropriate approach to the evaluation of global security than the state-centric extant theoretical frameworks employed in the study of international security. I describe the guiding principles behind the concept of human security and propose it as a new paradigm for studying international politics. I discuss the broad and integrative nature of this concept, some definitional and epistemological issues that pose a challenge to social scientific studies of human security, and the implications of this approach for global security. I present health as a core component of human security and provide a discussion of the linkages among human security, war, and public health.

Building on the discussion of human security, I present my conceptual and theoretical framework for studying the relationship between war and public health in Chapter 3. I present a brief overview of the literature on the consequences of conflict and point out the need for more comprehensive analyses of the effect of violent conflict on population well-being. Although significant scholarly efforts have been made to study the effects of conflict on states' political institutions and economic factors, far less has been done to understand the social consequences of conflict and the manner in which war can undermine the health of populations. I outline the key determinants of societies' health achievement, discuss my expectations for the direct and indirect ways in which conflict affects health, and explain the hypotheses that are tested in the empirical analyses in subsequent chapters. The chief influences on health examined in this book include violent international and internal conflict, general and health care infrastructure, economic resources, and forced migration.

Chapter 4 presents the first empirical analysis of the arguments made in Chapters 2 and 3. Specifically, it evaluates the effect of armed conflict on overall levels of health achievement in light of relevant political and economic factors. In this chapter, I address the questions of how levels of public health decline due to conflict in the short term and the long run, how national wealth affects health outputs, and how democracy is associated with population well-being. One important task at this stage is to appropriately define and measure public health. To this end, I rely heavily on the scholarship and methods of the discipline of public health. Most studies of population health use summary measures of public health that combine information on mortality and nonfatal health outcomes to express the health of a population as a single number, which includes inputs such as age-specific mortality and the epidemiology of nonfatal health outcomes. Murray et al. (2000) discuss these summary measures and claim that these measures are useful for comparing the health of different populations, comparing the health of the same population over time, and assessing the effects of nonfatal health outcomes on population health. I consult evaluations of summary health measures by public health scholars and choose Health-Adjusted Life Expectancy (HALE) as the most appropriate measure for the empirical analyses in this chapter. The statistical models demonstrate how conflict and other hypothesized influences affect overall health achievement in a universal sample of states from 1999 to 2002.

The summary measure of public health used in Chapter 4 is only available for the years 1999 to 2002. In Chapter 5, I extend the examination of the war-and-health relationship to a longer time period (from 1960 to 1999) using disaggregated measures of health achievement. These measures include male and female life expectancy, infant mortality rates, and fertility rates. I argue that conflict results in a deterioration of public health as measured by these indicators. Specifically, I expect that fertility rates and infant mortality rates to increase and life expectancies to decrease due to conflict, particularly as conflict duration increases. I also assess the effects of democracy, national income, trade openness, and population size on health indicators, and I evaluate regional differences in the relationship between war and health.

In Chapter 6, I examine one of the most important indirect mechanisms through which war undermines the well-being of populations: the destruction of key elements of societal infrastructure. I argue that both general infrastructure (such as transportation and power) and health care infrastructure (including hospitals and clinical facilities) are integral to the provision of adequate health care. Violent conflict has a direct and negative effect on all aspects of infrastructure, which in turn leads to a decline in health outputs. The empirical analysis focuses on the indirect effect of conflict—through infrastructure—on life expectancy, infant mortality, and fertility rates for the period from 1960 to 1999; the findings demonstrate strong linkages among war, infrastructure, and health.

I assess the relationship between the economic effect of war and health in Chapter 7. Here I examine the question of how the economic consequences of conflict affect public health and how resource allocation decisions during and after conflict have a detrimental effect on public health through budgetary trade-offs. States that become embroiled in conflict are often compelled to divert resources away from health expenditures (Mintz 1989) to meet the heightened needs for defense spending. War often results in economic decline and a decrease in overall resources available to a state, making it even more likely that fewer resources would be allocated to public health (Ward and Davis 1992). Discerning the effect of budgetary trade-offs on public health is crucial in evaluating the relationship between violence and health since violence can cause short- and long-term economic issues. I analyze empirically the relationships among war, national income, government spending, and public health for the period from 1970 to 2000; the analysis yields strong evidence for a negative effect of war on public health through economic decline and resource diversion.

Wars and violent conflicts often result in the generation of large refugee flows, and Chapter 8 explores the effect of forced migration on health achievement. Most of the direct and indirect effects of war on public health occur within the states in which the fighting takes place. The negative effects of refugee flows on health, however, are felt in the states to which these groups migrate. A large influx of refugees can lead to significant strains on a society's resources—including the health care system—and may, therefore, decrease a state's ability to meet the public health needs of its population. I argue that states that host large numbers of refugees will experience a decline in their health achievement, and I evaluate the linkages among war, forced migration, and health outputs for the period from 1965 to 1995.

Chapter 9 concludes the book with a discussion of the implications of my analyses of the relationship between war and health. I reiterate the importance of human security as a framework for understanding global security, the significance of health as an international issue, and the role of violent conflict as a determinant of national public health levels. I also discuss the importance of global involvement in conflict prevention and offer some future directions for research on the effect of violent conflict on health.

2

THE CONCEPT OF
HUMAN SECURITY

ASSESSING THE ADVERSE EFFECTS OF WAR on public health adds a new dimension to the study of conflict. It shifts the focus of analysis from the systemic or state level to the individual level (King and Martin 2001) as it evaluates the influence of conflict on the health of individuals in a society. It extends the idea of security from the security of states to the security of populations and fits well within the human security framework. Recently, scholars and policy makers have begun to focus attention on the issues of human security, including the effects of armed conflict on population well-being. For instance, King and Murray (2002) present a conceptualization of human security that takes into account health and economic factors rather than merely security from armed conflict. Their definition of human security focuses on the expected number of years of future life likely to be spent without falling "below the threshold of any key domain of human well-being" (585). This gives rise to the notion that public health is an important indicator of the level of human security enjoyed by the population of a state and, as I will demonstrate, public health is adversely affected by violent conflict. The first task at hand, therefore, is to understand the concept of human security. Although a number of varying and overlapping definitions of human security exist, it is appropriate to state that this concept focuses on the well-being and welfare of populations of states.

A PARADIGM OF HUMAN SECURITY?

There has been a growing awareness among policy-making and academic circles of the evolving nature of international security and the importance of population conditions in assessing global security. Although state security is by no means obsolete, it must be complemented by other elements of human security, including human rights and public health, to constitute fully the security of people. This calls for a "paradigm of security" (Commission on Human Security 2003) that takes into account threats to the well-being of individuals and communities that may not necessarily threaten state power. This view of security goes beyond the state-centric approach of traditional paradigms—such as realism—and implies the inclusion of actors other than just the state. In a speech in 2000, former United Nations (UN) Secretary-General Kofi Annan stated that "Human security, in its broadest sense, embraces far more than the absence of violent conflict. It encompasses human rights, good governance, access to education and health care and ensuring that each individual has opportunities and choices to fulfill his or her potential" (Annan 2000).

The human security framework was initially introduced in the 1994 *Human Development Report* of the United Nations Development Programme (UNDP), which called for a "profound transition in thinking . . . from nuclear security to human security" (22). During the Cold War, the concept of security had been limited to protecting territory, safeguarding national interests, and preventing a global nuclear war; hence, the notion of global security was closely associated with the territorial and political security of nation-states. The entire world was caught up in the tensions of the superpowers, the developed states striving to perpetuate their ideologies and the newly independent developing countries guarding themselves against any threats to their sovereignty. In the fray for military superiority, the plight of the ordinary people who populated sovereign states did not make it to the international relations agenda. As a result, both politics and scholarship were dominated by the realist paradigm, which emphasizes states as the key actors in the global system. What happened within the borders of states did not warrant international attention or action. Consequently, conflicts within states as well as the quality of life of individuals were relegated to domestic governance and received scarce attention from the international community, unlike interstate conflict.

The insecurity people suffered due to the threats of disease, famine, crime, economic decline, and repression was subordinated to the threat of military invasion. After the end of the Cold War, not only did the world community recognize the security menace posed by intrastate conflict, but it also became possible to turn attention to threats to the welfare of people within states. Clearly, state security is necessary for the security of people; however, state security alone does not bring about human security. The UNDP (1994) describes human security in negative terms:

> For most people, a feeling of insecurity arises more from worries about daily life than from the dread of a cataclysmic world event . . . human security is a child who did not die, a disease that did not spread, a job that was not cut, an ethnic tension that did not explode in violence, a dissident who was not silenced. Human security is not a concern with weapons—it is a concern with human life and dignity. (22)

Since human security deals with issues in the daily lives of people, there are two main elements of the concept. First, human security is safety from constant threats, such as repression and poverty, that prevent people from achieving a certain acceptable standard of living. Second, it is the absence of sudden catastrophic events that disrupt the lives of people, including natural disasters and war. The people-centric concept of human security is universal; the effects of threats such as environmental degradation, crime, drug trafficking, terrorism, and disease proliferation are not contained within any single state. The global nature of human security reflects the interdependence of the international community, and hence the threats to human security can best be addressed at the global level (United Nations Development Programme 1994).

The goal of human security is not to provide people with what they need for a comfortable life, but rather to enable people to better their own lives through adequate opportunities as well as to contribute to the development of society as a whole. Insecure people not only fail to enjoy a higher quality of life, but they also become a drain on the resources of their communities as social wards or miscreants. Secure individuals make secure societies, and secure societies make a secure global community. The UNDP (1994) listed seven components of human security: personal security, economic security, food security, health security, environmental security, community security, and political security. Personal security involves the ability of an individual to live his or her life without fear of physical harm to his or her person. Economic security, narrowly defined, refers to secure means for a basic income through productive work—hence, employment. Unemployment, and thus economic insecurity, can affect people in rich or poor states. Food security entails access to food at all times for every member of a society. This means that there is food available to be purchased at a reasonable price and that people have the economic means to buy food. Health security involves access to both preventive and curative health care, as well as protection from health threats, such as epidemics. Food and health security tend to be higher in developed states than in poorer countries. Environmental security entails safety from threats to the local as well as global ecosystems. Community security refers to the safety of groups, ranging from families to ethnic communities. People derive security from the groups to which they belong, and their security is threatened if those groups are persecuted or become involved in conflicts. Political security exists if the human and civil rights of people are respected by their states and members of societies do not suffer political repression. Based on these criteria, human security is a multifaceted concept that views population security through a holistic lens.

This early discussion of human security provides a framework for assessing the security needs of national and international communities in the post–Cold War era and highlights new dimensions of state vulnerabilities. The idea of human security represents a shift from realpolitik to a broader view of security in evaluating the state of the world, raising the responsibility of the international community from protecting the world from interstate or global war to protecting the people of the world. Although the idea that human security encompasses a number of threats to the lives of people is relatively new, the various components of human security are issues that have long been studied by various disciplines. Neither the academic world nor policy makers and practitioners are unfamiliar with problems such as poverty, environmental degradation, and disease. The human security framework merely presents an integrative approach to evaluating the welfare of people by reflecting the interconnectedness of these various issues. Since the initial discussion of human security in the 1994 UNDP report, there have been several attempts to refine the concept and explore its implications for academic research and political decision making. The growing emphasis on the study of human security reflects an awareness of the evolving nature of global security. The absence of interstate war is no longer sufficient for a secure world; global security can only be achieved through securing the populations of states. Important threats to the well-being and security of people—such as the HIV/AIDS epidemic, large-scale famine, and persistent poverty—in the current international system clearly demonstrate the significance of human security for global security.

The extant literature on human security offers a host of definitions for the concept and reveals the need to devote time and resources to developing a viable definitional and conceptual understanding of human security. Hampson and Hay (2003) examine the reasons for the rise of human security literature in the social sciences and suggest that academic work on the topic is merely proceeding some states' newfound emphasis on human security as a foreign policy priority. Canada and Japan are among such states. Establishments such as the Independent Commission on Human Security, along with the UN, are striving to launch a broader human security research agenda. The former UN Secretary-General, Kofi Annan, expressed a profound interest in issues of human security, including refugee conditions, racial discrimination, and women's rights. Practitioners in international conflict prevention, peacebuilding, human rights, and development have become increasingly cognizant of the need to comprehend and address human security needs. Consequently, students and scholars of conflict processes, public health, development, and other social scientific disciplines have begun exploring the implications of social, political, and economic phenomena for basic human needs.

Although it is easy to argue that human security is critical to global security, a major challenge to the study of human security is that there is no definitional or methodological consensus on the exact concept of human security. As the brief description of the UNDP (1994) definition of human security above illustrates, it is a broad concept with a range of interconnected components. The broad and multifaceted nature of the concept creates significant epistemological challenges in devising a precise definition and clear measurement of human security. Within the existing literature, three broad conceptions of human security can be identified (Hampson and Hay 2003). The first stems from liberal ideas of basic human rights and advocates notions of natural rights and the rule of law in determining the obligations of the international community in ensuring the security of people (Morsink 1998; Lauren 1998; Alston 1992). The second view of human security adheres to humanitarian considerations and calls for active intervention on the part of the international community in cases of human rights violations, such as genocide or atrocities during war (Boutros-Ghali 1992; Moore 1996). This second view is complementary to the first but calls for immediate and direct action by the international community and has led to extensive international activism as well as institutional involvement to combat violations of basic human rights. The third view of human security, which is the focus of this discussion, considers human security a much broader phenomenon that encompasses a large range of threats to the overall well-being and quality of life of individuals—including economic, environmental, and social menaces. There is ongoing debate between the merits of defining human security in broad terms of threats to human well-being and applying the term to the protection of a "limited vital core of human activities" that pertain to basic or fundamental human needs (Alkire 2002).

Protection from physical harm is indeed a core component of human security, but it does not adequately reflect the factors that enable people to lead secure lives. Although war is a devastating threat to the security of states and people, calamities such as famine, disease, and environmental contamination are also considerable impediments to human security. Consistent with the UNDP (1994) *Human Development Report*, Lodgaard (2000) argues that the end of the Cold War allowed for new perceptions of security as institutions and states were freed from the obsession with superpower conflict.

The Cold War subordinated national and international affairs to the logic of bloc politics. When the dictates of superpower rivalry were removed, the interests of governments and peoples came more clearly to the fore. Complex conflicts came into the open, and intra-state wars were waged with great ferocity. In this situation, the classical definition of security no longer sufficed. To retain its relevance to questions of war and peace, a companion concept to that of state security had to be introduced to cover the security of people as well. Defence could no longer be limited to the defence of state borders. It was also a matter of defending international rules, norms and standards in support of human beings at risk. (2)

The shift in perception of security from purely state-centric considerations to factors that influence populations of states is apparent in academic as well as policy circles. Securing the borders of states is important for the security of populations; however, that is far from a sufficient condition for ensuring the security of populations and, hence, human security.

Proponents of the broader view of human security are concerned with security in the lives of individuals, while traditional studies of international security focus on the security of states and consider war or invasion as the main security threat. Studying the phenomenon of security as the security of individuals—and by extension populations—is not to deprecate the magnitude of the impact of militarized violence on the political structure of states but to emphasize that secure borders are not synonymous with secure communities and secure people. The report of the Commission on Human Security (2003), *Human Security Now*, argues that human security complements state security by including threats that may not necessarily affect state security, encompassing issues of human rights and health care. It calls for an approach to human security that broadens the perceptions of security from state borders to people who live within the states. Threats to human security include environmental pollution, illiteracy, and ill health; for example, illness and lack of adequate health care caused more than 22 million preventable deaths in 2001 (Commission on Human Security 2003). Violent conflict, migration of refugees, and poverty-related issues such as economic deprivation represent a few of the negative influences on human security.

The emphasis in the human security debate on quality of life and welfare threats such as poverty, disease, hunger, and illiteracy reflect the importance of development. Ul Haq (1999) advocates looking at security through development instead of arms, and predicts a universal and indivisible perception of human security. He argues that it is "easier, more humane, and less costly to deal with the new issues of human security upstream rather than face their tragic consequences downstream" (80). Thakur (1997) emphasizes the importance of the quality of life of people as a core component of human security and views any challenges to their quality of life as threats to the security of people. Sen (2000) states that threats to human security include any menaces to the survival, daily life, and dignity of human beings; and McRae and Hubert (2002) call for a focus on the lives of individuals in evaluating the sociopolitical state of nations. Human security, however, cannot be viewed merely as a consequence or companion of development. Understanding the true nature of human security requires a holistic approach and attention to various influences on people's quality of life. According to the report of the Commission on Human Security (2003), the response of states and institutions to issues of human security "cannot be effective if it comes fragmented—from those dealing with rights, those with security, those with humanitarian concerns and those with development. With human security the objective, there must be a stronger and more integrated response from communities and states around the globe" (2). The breadth of human security as described by these ideas changes the focus of security from states to people as the object in need of security. It also shifts the burden of providing security from solely sovereign states to a number of actors, including governmental and nongovernmental institutions as well as national and local communities.

CRITICISM OF HUMAN SECURITY

The breadth of the concept of human security goes much further in capturing the state of populations than merely ascertaining the presence or absence of violent conflict. However, this breadth has also invited criticism on the basis of rendering the concept immeasurable. Paris (2001) criticizes existing definitions of human security for being "extraordinarily expansive and vague," failing to enable policy makers to form priorities on the bases of these definitions and leaving scholars unsure about the subject of study.

Paris states that proponents of human security perpetuate the vagueness of the concept by using "cultivated ambiguity" to rally support and use human security as a "campaign slogan." He argues that neither policy makers nor academics can benefit from this concept due to its inclusive nature. Descriptions of human security encompass such a large number of issues, ranging from personal freedom to global environment, that policy makers gain no insights into the need for focus on specific issues. The difficulty in deriving policy imperatives from the human security framework, he claims, arises due to the reluctance of human security advocates to prioritize issues. He considers treating all threats to security as equally important as one of the fundamental flaws of the concept of human security since this provides policy makers inadequate guidance in resource allocation decisions. Academics, Paris argues, are similarly unable to benefit from the concept of human security because the vagueness of the concept makes the subject to be examined unclear and hard to measure. Furthermore, causal relationships are difficult to identify due to the number of issues that constitute human security. Similarly, Mack (2001) argues that the broad definitions of the concept can make it difficult to keep the dependent and independent variables distinct in studies of human security. Thus the holistic and integrative qualities that make this approach ideal for studying world security also make it difficult to analyze in a social scientific manner.

Indeed, human security is a highly broad concept and does not lend itself to a single precise and simple definition. The breadth of the concept, however, does not necessarily render it vague, incomprehensible, or unable to be studied. In fact, human security has so far defied precise definition due to the complexity of the enterprise of including multiple issues into a single concept. The widely accepted individual threats to human security are salient and prevalent enough to warrant continued work in refining the concept rather than discarding it as a truism and shying away from further explorations of its definition and measurement. Further conceptual development of human security is a challenge rather than a futile exercise, and the ongoing work on the subject reflects the acceptance of that challenge.

The argument that the inclusiveness of human security does not provide policy makers any guidance for how to prioritize issues deprecates the ability of policy makers to discern the relative magnitude of the impact of various issues in their societies. As Paris (2001) asserts in his criticism, the concept of human security holds all threats to the security of people as equally important. However, proponents and scholars of the human security approach do not claim that all threats exist with the same intensity at all times in all states, warranting equal allocation of resources. In fact, the UNDP *Human Development Report* (1994) acknowledges that although the threats to human security are common to all people, "their intensity may differ from one part of the world to another" (22). For instance, hunger and access to health care are threats to the security of people in all states, but these threats are much more intense in poorer developing states than in the developed states of Western Europe and North America. Similarly, political repression is a major threat to human security in nondemocratic states. The relative intensity of the threats to human security in various states informs policy making by helping policy makers prioritize issues. The human security framework would suggest that a state that maintains adequate health care provisions but suffers from high levels of unemployment needs to allocate more resources to the stimulation of the economy and creation of jobs; a repressive state that violates the human rights of its population calls for intervention by the international community. Krause and Williams (1996) suggest that broad ideas of security inform policies for eliminating security threats:

> It may be necessary to broaden the agenda of security studies (theoretically and methodologically) in order to narrow the agenda of *security*. A more profound understanding of the forces that create political loyalties, give rise to threats, and designate appropriate collective responses could open the way to . . . the progressive removal of issues from the security agenda as they are dealt with via institutions and practices that do not implicate force, violence, or the "security dilemma." There is nothing inevitable or idealistic about this idea. Contemporary political debates over the enlargement of NATO, the appropriate preventive responses to nascent communal conflicts, and the imperatives of dealing with rapid environmental change all suggest that policy makers engage daily with the complexities and possibilities of "security" in a broad sense. (249)

The purpose of human security as a concept is to provide policy makers with a framework to assess the needs of their individual societies and to identify major societal vulnerabilities, rather than to compel them to allocate equal resources to all threats to security.

The issue of measurement is a more plausible problem in the study of human security. The inclusion of a large number of human security threats makes it difficult to derive a precise single measure of the phenomenon and creates the methodological issue of unclear delineation between human security as the dependent variable and the independent variables that influence its levels. Scholars are working toward formulating viable measures of human security. For instance, King and Murray (2002) present a model that uses poverty, health, education, political freedom, and democracy as key components of human security. That, however, raises the issue of how to decide which of the many issues related to human security go into the measure. The methodological challenges associated with the study of human security are real, but the importance of the concept for the well-being of societies necessitates continued research. Although no single undisputed measure of human security exists, the individual components of—or threats to—human security are measurable and widely studied. Even in the absence of a single measure, human security has the potential to reshape scholarship on security by broadening the field to include social, economic, environmental, and other factors.

Human security is useful to scholars and policy makers as an overarching framework within which social scientific studies are conducted that focus on narrower issues. The issue of accurate measurement does not eliminate the relevance of human security as a conceptual shift in the study of security. Measurement issues become less relevant if human security—as many of its proponents suggest—is viewed as a paradigm rather than a phenomenon. In this book, I employ this paradigm by focusing on violent conflict as a threat to human security and by assessing the effect of war on the health of societies. This study thus deviates from traditional analyses of the consequences of war and is consistent with the concept of human security, in that it evaluates the effect of conflict on people and not merely on states.

WAR AND HUMAN SECURITY

The human security framework does not view war and violent conflict as the only threats to security and the state as the only object whose security is important. However, that is not to say that it deprecates the significance of violent conflict for the security of people. Conflict affects states as well as the people within states, and students of human security are concerned with the manner in which conflict influences the well-being of populations. Violent conflict, including wars and terrorism, undermines the security of people by causing large-scale death and destruction as well as by adversely affecting their quality of life. Civil wars and interstate conflicts destroy cities and cause deaths; people are subjected to human rights violations and forced to leave their homes. Even if people do not suffer these immediate effects of war, their daily lives are affected through generalized insecurity, poverty, or hopelessness. The concept of human security does not imply that the relevance of violent conflict as a security threat has diminished; it asserts that violence needs to be studied as a threat to the security of people rather than just the security of states.

Between 1990 and 2001, there were 57 major armed conflicts in 45 countries; there were 24 armed conflicts in 2001 alone, most of which occurred in Africa (Commission on Human Security 2003). The majority of recent armed conflicts have been internal and have led to serious consequences, including state failure and economic collapse. In addition to domestic consequences, these conflicts have had repercussions for their neighboring states since other states in the region often tend to become involved in civil strife, as in the case of the Democratic Republic of Congo. Hence the effects of conflict are becoming increasingly difficult to contain within the borders of individual states. In addition to state-level conflicts, transnational organized crime and terrorism networks cause a decrease in human security. Terrorism generates insecurity in people and impedes their ability to lead normal lives without fear. The strength of terrorist organizations in any state is a threat to global security as terrorist networks continue to become increasingly internationalized. The global nature of threats such as terrorism requires an international commitment to the protection of human security.

Armed conflict also affects the lives of people by forcing them to leave their homes and migrate. In 2000, there were 16 million refugees in the world and more than 25 million people internally displaced due to violent conflict, domestic violence, or human rights abuses (Commission on Human Security 2003). Large refugee flows can create security and social issues for host states as well. The refugee population can be a strain on the resources of the host state, which could compel the host to close its borders. Recent concerns with terrorism have also led to tighter controls on refugee flows. As a result, many people are incapable of escaping conflict-ridden states. Refugee flows and internal displacement further decrease human security by causing economic deprivation, violence within the migrant groups, and spread of infectious diseases like HIV/AIDS.

Many threats to human security emerge after conflict has officially ceased. A peace settlement or official cessation of hostilities between warring parties might represent security at the state level, but it rarely ensures security for the people. Violent conflict may impose millions of dollars worth of damage on a society and cause people years' worth of labor. This damage, combined with the depletion of economic resources during the conflict, often makes it tremendously difficult for societies to recover from war. Since most recent armed conflicts have been in some of the world's poorest states, the ability of societies to rebuild after conflict is severely limited. Moreover, peace following a settlement does not always last and violence often resumes after a while, as in the case of several African conflicts, making rebuilding impossible (Bigombe et al. 2000). Recurrent armed conflict may be accompanied by increases in interpersonal violence and crime. It is important, therefore, for the international community to make a commitment to assist states in post-conflict recovery and reconstruction in order to mitigate the lingering effects of conflict on human security. International intervention, however, varies widely among conflicts and ranges from extensive and lasting involvement, as in the former Yugoslavia, to a complete lack of international interest, as in Armenia and Azerbaijan. If the goals of human security are to be met at the global level, international actors need to make a commitment to post-conflict political, economic, and social recovery in all affected states. The traditional approach to security would consider a state secure once a war or conflict has ended, at which point international intervention is no longer required. The concept of human security, on the other hand, argues that security has not been achieved until the population of the conflict-ridden society has completely recovered. This approach prodigiously increases the obligations of the international community and domestic leadership. During the conflict, efforts are to be made to protect civilian populations and to provide humanitarian aid, including food and health care, to those who need it. Conditions that promote refugee flows and internal displacement are to be prevented; failing that, migrant groups and their hosts are to be assisted in meeting their security needs. After the fighting ends, it becomes important to ascertain that the population is physically safe and that people's basic needs are met. Security of people also entails the establishment of stable political institutions, economic recovery, proper law enforcement, prevention of various forms of violence, and large-scale rehabilitation and reconstruction. Violent conflict truly highlights the need for a human security approach, as it has the potential to heighten nearly all of the threats to human security.

HEALTH AND HUMAN SECURITY

Most definitions of human security include health as an integral component of the security of people. Since the very purpose of human security is to protect human lives and people's quality of life, health is undeniably a necessary condition for human security, and illness, disease, disability, and high mortality rates are serious threats to human security. Good health provisions include prevention of infectious diseases as well as availability of treatment for ailments and accidental illness. The last century has witnessed remarkable advancements in health care and medical sciences. Improvements in medical provisions, scientific research, and increased production of food have led to high life expectancies in most of the world. However, the positive effects of these advancements are by no means equitably distributed among the nations of the world; there are immense differences in the level of health and longevity in different states.

Poverty and conflict are closely related to health; for instance, the average life expectancies in Sierra Leone and Ethiopia are about half of the average life expectancies in Japan and Sweden (United Nations Development Programme 2002). There are nearly 56 million deaths every year and 40 percent of these deaths would be avoidable with adequate access to medical resources (World Health Organization 2003). Many of these avoidable deaths occur in communities that live in poverty or are in conflict-ridden regions; for instance, HIV/AIDS rates are significantly higher in sub-Saharan Africa than in any other region of the world. The average rate of HIV/AIDS prevalence in sub-Saharan Africa is 7.4 percent, which is drastically higher than the rates of 0.6 percent in North America, Latin America, and in South and East Asia (Iqbal and Zorn 2010). Most of the states of sub-Saharan Africa also suffer from poverty and protracted conflict.

The Commission on Human Security (2003) states that three major health challenges are closely related to human security: poverty-related health issues, infectious diseases, and violence:

> Most preventable infectious diseases, nutritional deprivation and maternity-related risks are concentrated among the world's poor. Poverty and disease set up a vicious spiral with negative economic and human consequences. And all forms of violence— collective, interpersonal and self-directed—are public health problems. Indeed, the growing social crises of violence all have strong health dimensions. (98)

Similar to many other threats to human security, health-related issues can have a global dimension. Infectious diseases and epidemics cannot be contained within state borders. Increased travel makes the spread of disease—as well as treatment resistance—across countries and regions extremely rapid and dangerous. This danger has amply been demonstrated by public health crises such as outbreaks of mad cow disease and SARS. The spread of HIV/AIDS to practically every part of the world also reflects the global nature of disease and the seriousness of the problem of disease proliferation. Although disease does not recognize state borders, infectious diseases tend to be more prevalent among poorer communities due to malnutrition, lack of clean water and sanitation, lack of access to preventive health care and immunizations, and environmental threats.

The human security approach to health demands that people are protected from disease by eliminating the conditions that might lead to preventable illness and death. Fulfillment of economic needs, better environmental conditions, lack of violence, literacy, plentiful food, and clean water are all necessary conditions for good health and human security. These conditions would empower people to maintain adequate levels of personal health and free social institutions from the burden of caring for large numbers of ailing individuals. Moreover, adequate medical provisions for prevention and treatment of disease and disability are essential for security through health. This, in turn, necessitates policy decisions that allocate sufficient resources to social spending and public health. At the global level, involvement of international institutions in promoting good health through dissemination of information and development of global surveillance systems would contribute to better health conditions. The global community must be prepared to engage in immediate action for health emergencies—such as spread of epidemics, as well as long-term disease surveillance and monitoring. The health threats to human security can only be ameliorated if action is taken at the individual, local, national, and global levels.

THE IMPLICATIONS OF HUMAN SECURITY

The main goal of the human security agenda is to bring about an evolution in security priorities whereby human security is placed on the top in decision making at the global, regional, national, and local levels. This would entail integrating concerns related to development, human rights, and a number of other issues. The purposes of focusing on human security are to prevent conflict, advance development, improve human rights, protect people, spread and strengthen democracy, and promote a culture of human security.[1] Human security stresses the cost of conflict for people, thus making it important to facilitate conflict prevention. Measures such as diplomatic efforts, early warning mechanisms, peacekeeping missions, and transparency become more important if human security—rather than military superiority—is dictating foreign policy. At the domestic level, establishment of civil society, democracy, political freedom, and education can contribute to conflict prevention through political participation and checks on power. Economic well-being and political security diminish dissatisfaction among individuals and groups, reducing the likelihood of political violence and civil strife. By recognizing the security needs of people along with those of states, human security encourages policies for "minimizing risks, adopting preventive measures to reduce human vulnerabilities and taking remedial action when prevention fails" (Bruderlein 2001, 358).

Policies driven by human security would ensure the protection of people at the national and international levels. This would be reflected in effective institutions at various levels—including health care networks, education systems, law enforcement agencies, and environmental regulations. Successful functioning of such institutions would lead to enabling people to act on their own behalves and improve their own quality of life. Democracy is an important aspect of the empowerment of people; democratic principles allow people to voice their grievances, participate in governance, and mobilize to protect their interests. Hence, democracy is one of the most important steps in ensuring human security as it empowers people and strengthens institutions. Human security invites the involvement of state and non-state actors in enhancing the security of people. Bruderlein (2001) argues for the effectiveness of non-state actors in tackling issues of human security:

> The measures required to enhance human security often call for action from numerous non-state actors, particularly NGOs, in addressing, for example, the needs of the displaced populations, advocating stronger control over the arms trade or assisting governments in preserving and restoring fragile environments. Human security can serve as a platform to call on non-state actors, along with states, to help in dealing with the causes of global insecurity. (360)

Human security aims to cultivate integration across issues, geographical divisions, and the range of actors. Since the threats to human security emerge from many directions and take varying forms, no one actor, such as the state, is suited singled-handedly to address those issues.

In the academic realm, the human security framework aims to refine the perception of security and broaden the scope of issues addressed by students and scholars of security. Human security suggests a research agenda that scientifically assesses the influences on the security of people across a range of disciplines, including political science, economics, sociology, and public health. Studies informed by this framework would deal with a wide spectrum of factors affecting societal well-being and employ the theories and methodologies offered by relevant academic disciplines to conduct theoretical and empirical research. Future directions for research on human security include the development of better measurements for human security and its components. To date, there is no coherent index that measures the security of populations. Moreover, continued work on the assessment of various threats to human security is required in order to better understand the concept. This book furthers the goals of human security by providing a social scientific evaluation of the effect of conflict on health and offering a clearer understanding of the costs of war in terms of population security.

CONCLUSION

The perception of human security as a complex combination of numerous elements that contribute to a secure life for the populations of states, including but not limited to the power of sovereign states, reflects the importance of studying the influences on the health of societies. Provision of adequate public health is a significant element of the security and well-being of populations and could be heavily influenced by states' involvement in war. Is a society secure if its population does not enjoy adequate health care? Are populations safe from the impact of violent conflict if they are able to escape the immediate devastation of combat? Or does war have indirect effects on the health and quality of life of people? Considering the mechanisms through which militarized conflict undermines human security at various levels— such as the effect on public health—emphasizes the need for studying the consequences of war beyond the termination of hostilities among states or settlements of civil wars. Even after the actual war has ended and settlements have been made among leaderships of states or groups, the populations of those states may continue to face threats to their security. The analyses in this book employ the human security framework to examine the relationship between war and population health and the effect of violent conflict on the security of people. The next chapter outlines the theoretical argument of the study and relevant hypotheses about the relationship between conflict and the health of populations. Subsequent chapters present empirical tests for these arguments.

3

War and Health: A Conceptual and Theoretical Framework

IN CHAPTER 2, I outlined the relevance of human security as an appropriate framework to assess the security of people as well as global security. The concept of human security asserts that global security can truly be achieved only through the security of people, for which state security is a necessary but not sufficient condition. Human security calls for an integrative approach in assessing the security needs of populations, taking into account a host of socioeconomic factors that might pose threats to people's quality of life—such as poverty, disease, war, repression, and environmental hazards. Public health is an undisputed component of human security, which I examine in the context of violent conflict.

War results in direct and indirect negative effects on public health. The immediate and direct effects of war include military and civilian casualties; large numbers of people are killed or wounded during combat. However, the impact of conflict on the health of societies does not end there; involvement in conflict leads to conditions that make it difficult for states to meet their health care needs, such as damage to health care facilities, diversion of medical resources and personnel to defense purposes, and issues of health care accessibility due to disruptions in transportation and communications. Moreover, wars are often associated with increased health care needs due to combat-related injuries and the spread of infectious diseases. Destruction of infrastructure, movement of people, malnutrition, and lack of clean water are some of the factors that contribute to the proliferation of disease during and after a war. The effect of conflict on health is an important and highly detrimental consequence of war to which scholars have not paid much attention. In this chapter, I present the conceptual framework within which I assess the effect of conflict on health. First, I offer an overview of the literature on the consequences of conflict. Next, I lay out the theory and hypotheses of this study. And then I briefly discuss the implications of this work for human security.

THE CONSEQUENCES OF CONFLICT

Research on the relationship between violent conflict and public health contributes to a better understanding of the determinants of human security, elucidates the human cost of war, and contributes to the burgeoning theoretical and empirical literature on the consequences of conflict. Scholars have long been interested in the cost of waging war and the economics of defense spending (Russett 1969, 1970; Stewart and Fitzgerald 2001), and more recently there has been a growing literature on the consequences of conflict. The literature on the political consequences of war explores issues such as democratization, political institutions, leaders and regime type, international power, and human rights (Bueno de Mesquita and Siverson 1995, 1997; Bueno de Mesquita et al. 1992; Rasler and Thompson 1985). Work on the termination of war addresses issues regarding settlements following conflict, reconstruction, and peacekeeping (Werner 1998, 1999; Walter 1999), as well as the fate of leaders after a conflict (Goemans 2000a, 2000b). Bueno de Mesquita et al. (1992) explore the question of whether the decision to go to war results in violent removal of a state's leadership and argue that "a failed policy in the domain of international war will render a regime vulnerable to removal" (640). They find that the well-being of a regime is strongly tied to its performance in war. Leaderships that impose heavy war costs on their states are likely to be deposed. The negative effect of war on leadership duration is further demonstrated by Bueno de Mesquita and Siverson (1995): "those leaders who subject their nations to war subject themselves to a political hazard that threatens the very essence of the office holding *homo politicus*—the retention of political power" (852). Hence, war can result in the end of a regime, possibly in a way that causes domestic political upheaval.

Conflict also influences democratization, though the literature is mixed as to how conflict hinders the process of democratization. Involvement in conflict or aspirations for territorial conquests facilitate a political atmosphere in which the development of democracy is stifled. Thompson (1996) argues for a reverse causation in the democracy-peace relationship. In his analysis of partially democratic regions, he finds that:

> (1) democratization was facilitated by states being forced to abandon their aspirations to regional hegemony, choosing not to pursue regional hegemony, or some combination; (2) states in the process of becoming more democratic and that also found themselves pursuing regional hegemony suppressed the former process in favor of the latter; or (3) states that became more democratic did so in part because their regions were not characterized by extensive interstate conflict in the first place. (147)

Mitchell et al. (1999) disagree with Thompson about the long-term impediment to democracy posed by warfare; they argue that the negative effect of war on democracy might exist in the short run, but the overall effect of war is to cause democratic transitions. Mousseau and Shi (1999) evaluate the relationship between war and democracy as anterior, concurrent, and posterior effects and do not find strong evidence for reverse causality in democratic peace; they caution against letting the reverse causality arguments make democracy irrelevant as a viable explanation for peace. Reiter (2001) finds that "only the highest level of international conflict—current participation in international war—significantly reduces the chances that a state will make the transition to democracy" (944). Involvement in lower levels of conflict, such as interventions, does not decrease the possibility of democratization; nor does war result in autocratic transitions of democracies (Reiter 2001).

While some scholars have demonstrated that conflict has significant political costs and consequences, others have concentrated on the economic effects of conflict (e.g., Organski and Kugler 1980). Rasler and Thompson

(1983, 1985) evaluate the short-term and long-term impacts of different types of conflict on economic growth. They find that although the economic effects of most interstate wars are temporary, the more intensive wars that they term "global wars" tend to have significant long-term deleterious economic effects. Collier (1999) discusses the economic consequences of conflict and argues that there could be a "war overhang" effect of civil wars on GDP growth rate. Conflict destroys the economic resources and disrupts the economic activity of the state. Consequently, the GDP plummets suddenly in the short run and the GDP growth rate continues to be affected after the war is over. Fitzgerald (2001) argues that some of the worst indirect costs of conflict arise from macroeconomic disequilibria caused by hyperinflation, decrease in real wages, and shortages in supplies of goods and services.

Stewart and Fitzgerald (2001) discuss underdevelopment as an important consequence of war and criticize existing work on development for neglecting war as a cause of poverty and a hindrance to development, "although countries which have suffered civil war account for eight out of the ten countries with the highest infant mortality rates and of those with the lowest per capita incomes" (3). They examine the vulnerability of an economy to the effects of war and suggest that factors such as per-capita income, poverty levels, trade dependence, and the adaptability of the production system, influence how an economy responds to war. More importantly, however, the nature of the war determines its economic effects:

> The economic consequences are clearly highly dependent on the nature of the war itself. Most obviously, the duration of the war is an important element. In a long war, reserves will be exhausted, so vulnerability is increased. However, people will have more time to adapt their lifestyles to the war context, and so protect their productivity and living standards. The geographic spread of the war is also important. When confined to one part of the country the war may have only small direct effects on the economy as a whole, thus reducing national vulnerability, although where war expenditures are high in relation to the resources of a state, the indirect social costs can become very large, increasing vulnerability. The extent of foreign involvement in the war is another factor affecting vulnerability, since external support may compensate for lost export earnings. (9)

The interactions between war and the economy are complex and numerous, bearing strong influences on the short-term well-being of an economic structure as well as the long-term development prospects of a society.

The devastating effects of war include the creation of environmental hazards that can lead to long-term consequences for a society.[2] During the Gulf War, Iraq employed environmental destruction as a weapon and set fire to numerous oil wells in Kuwait. The fires that burned for about ten months resulted in smoke clouds throughout the region and severe air pollution. Dickie and Gerking (2000) attempt to measure the value of the damage caused by the environmental devastation of the Gulf War and claim that it represents one of the worst environmental catastrophes in recorded history. Environmental damage adversely affects human health through air pollution, water pollution, and indirectly through its effects on agriculture. Leaning (1999) also demonstrates that conflict leads to detrimental environmental consequences, which in turn carry repercussions for the public health of the society. She discusses the environmental hazards arising from the activities of the Cold War, such as production and testing of nuclear weapons, use of land mines, and storage of military waste. The rising awareness of the environmental consequences of conflict and their impact on public health reflects the importance of examining public health in the context of war.

In addition to the political, economic, and environmental impacts of conflict, war results in a host of social consequences as well. The effect on the health of a society is a core component of the social consequences of conflict, and a much more profound understanding of this consequence is required. A number of linkages among conflict, its social consequences, and public health remain to be explored. Studying the effect of war on health explores an important consequence of conflict in light of the human security framework, which goes beyond state-level factors and considers myriad elements that constitute the security of populations. Although a few attempts have been made to assess the public health impact of various forms of armed conflict, this area of research remains underdeveloped. In the next section, I discuss some of the extant works on the relationship between various forms of armed conflict and public health.

CONFLICT AND HEALTH

In this book, I answer some important questions raised by the nascent literature on the public health consequences of conflict by exploring the causal mechanisms involved in the effects of war on health. This study demonstrates the suitability of this subject within the international relations literature and provides a more lucid basis for understanding the war-health relationship for policy makers and practitioners in public health and humanitarian endeavors. The effect of conflict on states has extensively been studied and the theoretical and methodological tools offered by existing literature can be used to examine the consequences of conflict for the civilian populations of war-torn states. The existing literature on conflict and public health (for example, King and Murray 2002; King and Martin 2001; Ghobarah et al. 2003, 2004) has made valuable contributions to modeling linkages between health and conflict and has raised some interesting questions about the relationship between the two phenomena. However, this literature lacks the specificity needed to understand fully the relationship between conflict and population well-being. The relationship between conflict and public health is a topic of great concern to political scientists as well as to scholars in other disciplines that are concerned with population issues—including economics, sociology, and public health; yet social scientific literature evaluating this relationship remains limited.

To the extent that empirical analyses of the effect of violent conflict on population health have been undertaken, the existing research highlights important linkages between war and health and opens the door to a range of future directions for research in the area. In one such study, Ghobarah et al. (2003) conduct a cross-national analysis using political and economic variables to assess the relationship between conflict and public health and emphasize the role of public health in human security. Their study employs summary measures of public health to illustrate the linkages between political factors, such as conflict, and the quality of public health in a society; their findings show a clearly negative relationship between violent conflict and public health even after a conflict has ended. Specifically, they find that the burden of death and disability in 1999, from the effects of conflicts between 1991 and 1997, was nearly the same as the direct fatal and nonfatal health effects that occurred immediately from all the violent conflicts in 1999. In another study of war and health, Davis and Kuritsky (2002) find that sub-Saharan countries that were involved in military conflict between 1968 and 1999 experienced lower life expectancies and higher infant mortality rates than sub-Saharan countries that were not involved in conflict. Particularly, as Pedersen (2002) asserts, contemporary wars have stronger repercussions for the physical and mental health of populations than wars in the past due to the strategic use of health personnel and facilities. For instance, during the conflict between the Mozambican National Resistance (RENAMO) guerrillas and the Mozambique government forces, 1,000 health centers were destroyed and land mines were placed near hospitals. In addition to the direct and indirect effects on physical health conditions, war also causes trauma-related mental health issues, including anxiety, depression, and drug abuse (Pedersen 2002).

The developing literature on war and population well-being raises a host of questions about the mechanisms through which conflict affects health, as well as issues of conceptualization and measurement. Ghobarah et al. (2003) effectively set the stage for my study; they use a summary measure, Disability-Adjusted Life Years (DALY), as the dependent variable for assessing the effect of civil wars on public health. The DALY measure reflects "the life-years lost due to deaths from a particular condition . . . plus the expected disability to be incurred by other people who suffered from the same condition in that same year" (190). This measure is derived from the Health-Adjusted Life Expectancy (HALE) measure, which was previously known as the Disability-Adjusted Life Expectancy (DALE) measure. The next chapter discusses summary measures of health, particularly HALE, in greater detail. The DALY measure is different from HALE/DALE in that it breaks down the effect of disability and disease into gender and five age groups and attributes deaths to certain causes. Although the aggregation of data by disease and population groups makes DALYs more informative in some ways, the measure is only available for 1999, which is the year to which the Ghobarah et al. (2003) study is limited. Ghobarah et al. (2003) briefly touch upon the relationships among civil war, resource allocation, and refugee migration. However, their cursory treatment of these issues begs for further exploration of the strong linkages among various consequences of conflict. I conduct a more in-depth analysis of the mechanisms through which conflict affects health, taking into account all kinds of militarized conflict and analyzing some important issues in the conflict-health relationship, such as budgetary trade-offs.

In another work, Ghobarah et al. (2004) examine the effect of public and private spending on levels of public health. They employ the DALE measure for 1999 in that analysis, which imposes the same temporal limitation as the analysis discussed above. Their argument about the negative effect of war on health due to economic influences is consistent with one of the arguments I present in this study, stating that economic decline and resource diversion caused by war can negatively affect public health. Chapter 7 addresses this argument, and while Ghobarah et al. (2004) limit their analysis to civil wars, I include all instances of armed conflict that reached a certain threshold of violence. Ghobarah et al. (2004) assert that "civil wars reduce the productivity of the entire economy, and especially damage and disrupt the administrative and economic infrastructure necessary to maintain previous levels of health expenditure" (15). As public spending on health decreases during long conflicts, they argue, private spending on health care rises. Consequently, there may not be any noticeable difference in health expenditure due to involvement in conflict (Ghobarah et al. 2004). Their findings suggest, however, that public spending may in fact increase during a civil war, with no effect on health spending if a neighboring state is experiencing civil war.

The research examining the relationship between violent conflict and public health levels remains scarce, and an even smaller body of literature examines the reverse causality in this relationship. A few scholars have examined the pernicious effects of disease and other health threats on national security, particularly the influence of HIV/AIDS rates on violent conflict. Elbe (2002, 2003), for instance, analyzes the effect of the HIV/AIDS epidemic on the behavior of armed forces in African conflicts and the impact of the disease on broader social, political, and economic factors. He argues that high rates of HIV prevalence among combatants reduce their military effectiveness, which in turn decreases state security. Moreover, since they serve as vectors for the spread of the disease, prevalence of the disease raises the social costs of the conflict. By emphasizing that "the AIDS pandemic should be understood not only as a global health issue but also as an international security issue" (Elbe 2002, 176), he calls attention to the need to study the effect of the disease on violent conflict. Elbe (2003) proposes a positive relationship between increasing numbers of AIDS orphans and violent conflict and civil unrest. Peterson and Shellman (2006) conduct an empirical analysis of the effect of HIV/AIDS on the levels of state-imposed human rights violations and violent intrastate conflict. They find that, although HIV rates do not have a direct effect on human rights abuses and domestic conflict, they do undermine national security through the deterioration of social, political, and economic institutions of a state. Price-Smith (2001, 2003, 2009) and Price-Smith and Daly (2004) examine a number of dimensions of the negative effect of infectious disease, particularly HIV/AIDS, on aspects of national security. For instance, Price-Smith (2009) argues that epidemics challenge the security of a state through the deterioration of its power, since widespread disease may lead to domestic political instability; furthermore, there may be a negative effect on a state's international relations. Similarly, Ostergard (2002) calls attention to the need to study HIV/AIDS in Africa as a security threat, arguing for instance that "extended periods of illness and finally death of policy makers can render decision making inconsistent" (341) and that "the virus has the potential to compromise military performance because of the chance for opportunistic infections to appear as a result of soldiers' weakened immune systems" (344).

Although there are some salient questions regarding the effects of disease and low public health levels on national and international security, the purpose of this book is to examine the manner in which violent conflict influences the degree of health and well-being enjoyed by a population. The primary concern in the study of human security is assessment of threats to, and determinants of, population well-being. As I have stated earlier, public health lies at the core of human security and armed conflict poses an obviously serious—but understudied—threat to the health outputs of a society; and that is the relationship that I analyze in this book. To the extent that a decline in population health may be demonstrated to reduce international security, it further emphasizes the importance of understanding and mitigating negative influences on societal well-being.

With respect to the existing literature on the social and public health consequences of violent conflict, that work serves to present many interesting questions and empirical puzzles. However, extant research falls short of offering a comprehensive theoretical exploration or conducting an exhaustive empirical study of the relationship between conflict and public health. Several analyses demonstrate that a relationship exists between violent conflict and population health and that conflict adversely affects health outcomes, but this relationship needs to be subjected to more thorough analysis to better explain the effect of conflict on the well-being of societies. Moreover, a lack of exhaustive data has limited the scope of research on the topic. Further theoretical as well as empirical work is called for in the examination of the social and health consequences of violent conflict, and this book contributes toward that goal. Below I present the conceptual and theoretical framework that I employ in the analysis of the relationship between war and health.

THEORY AND HYPOTHESES

There have been a few studies that look at conflict and public health but these studies do not thoroughly examine the relevant linkages. Violent conflict may affect public health through damage to the infrastructure of the society, both by interrupting access to basic services such as water and transportation and by limiting availability of health care personnel. Economic resources get diverted from public health to military uses and the environmental damage resulting from conflict gives rise to disease. Strong linkages exist among the more obvious consequences of war—such as the toll on the environmental and economic well-being of a society—and the health consequences of violent conflict. Conflict also generates refugee flows; the living conditions of refugees are generally not conducive to good health and refugees can transmit disease across borders (Ghobarah et al. 2003).

By looking at history, it is clear that war influences public health beyond the direct casualties of combat. For instance, the influenza epidemic that spread in 1918 and 1919 killed more people than the deaths that resulted directly from military activity in World War I. Estimates of deaths due to the 1918 influenza epidemic range from 20 to 40 million; the epidemic started in Europe but very quickly reached global proportions. Approximately 675,000 Americans died of the disease, with outbreaks all over North America, Asia, Africa, Europe, South America, and the Pacific (Taubenberger 1997). The origins of the virus remain unknown, but some of the causes of the magnitude that the epidemic reached included the mass movements of armed forces, the conditions in which soldiers lived in the trenches, and the effects of mustard gas and fumes generated by some weapons.

Conditions in the war-affected areas of Europe during World War I were ripe for the spread of infection; mobility of soldiers and people aboard ships transported the virus to regions not involved in the war. The effect of the disease was aggravated by the inability of medical facilities and personnel to meet the needs of the afflicted, particularly the civilians. Most physicians and other trained medical personnel were mobilized for the treatment of troops with nonfatal battle injuries or contracted the influenza themselves. This public health catastrophe revealed that the human cost of war can reach far beyond the numbers of battle deaths. It demonstrated that war simultaneously facilitates conditions in which public health emergencies arise and reduces the capabilities of societies to meet their health needs. Further, health threats cannot be contained within a state or a region and can rapidly reach global dimensions.

More recently, the negative effect of war on health was clearly manifested by disruption of health care provisions in Iraq due to the 1991 Gulf War. The civilian population of Iraq was severely affected by the devastation of the war due to destruction of infrastructure, breakdown of communications, incapacitation of the transportation system, lack of food and medical supplies, and proliferation of disease. According to the World Health Organization Division of Emergency and Humanitarian Action (1998a):

> The six-week war in 1991 resulted in the destruction of a large number of public health facilities in Iraq (electricity plants, water purification plants, health infrastructure, etc.), disrupting partially or completely provisions for regular health services. The sanctions imposed on Iraq since 1990 impeded the country from: repairing damaged or destroyed infrastructure, continuing regular health programmes, importing

at necessary levels vital goods such as food and medicine. . . . Assessment missions report that the quality of health care in Iraq has regressed by at least 50 years. Diseases such as malaria, typhoid and cholera, which were once almost under control, have rebounded since 1991 at epidemic levels.

The combination of the havoc wreaked by attacks during the war and postwar sanctions left the Iraqi health care system in shambles. The situation was made worse by increased health care needs of the population due to the casualties of war and conditions that led to deteriorating health outcomes, such as lack of adequate food supplies and skyrocketing inflation.

Child mortality in Iraq increased from 257 per 100,000 in 1990 to 1,536 per 100,000 in 1995 (World Health Organization 1998a). Before the war, 90 percent of the Iraqi population had access to health care, with high standards of hospital facilities, medical staff, and laboratory support. After the war, laboratory services declined by approximately 50 percent and medical supplies became severely limited. The hospitals that continued to function after the war provided unsanitary and overcrowded facilities that did just as much to spread infections as they did to treat ailments. The entire city of Baghdad did not have access to clean water or sanitation, causing rampant spread of infectious diseases. The incidence of typhoid cases, for example, went up from 11.3 per 100,000 people in 1990 to 142.1 per 100,000 people in 1994 (World Health Organization 1998a). The immediate impact of war on health was exacerbated by the Iraqi society's inability to rebuild and recover after the war due to sanctions and lack of economic resources.

These examples reflect how militarized conflict affects the public health of a population at several levels. The direct effects of conflict include the number of people killed and wounded in the conflict. But conflict also affects public health through exposure of populations to hazardous conditions caused by activities such as refugee flows and movement of soldiers, giving rise to epidemics as the mobile groups act as vectors for disease. The ability of war-torn societies to deal with new threats to public health is weakened by conflict and, consequently, the negative effect on health outcomes continues to grow. Public health provisions go below prewar levels and demands on the health care system rise above prewar levels. Consequently, large numbers of people may be left without appropriate health care and, even for those who have access to health care facilities, the quality of health care provisions may be lower than before the war. Access to adequate health care could be particularly difficult for the civilian population if treatment of military casualties takes precedence over the health care needs of civilians.

During periods of conflict, resources get diverted toward military purposes and public health spending may be reduced, even as the public health needs of the population escalate. This diversion of resources away from public health is often accompanied by a decline in infrastructure that further impedes the ability of a society to handle the society's health care demands. Damage to the general infrastructure combines with damage to or possible destruction of the health care infrastructure to make a society incapable of facing its increasing public health challenges. The health of the population is affected not only by direct damage to hospitals and other medical facilities, but also by damage to elements of the larger infrastructure such as transportation, the water supply, and power grids. At a more indirect level, conflict may lead to a general social and economic decline that has dire long-term consequences for the health of a society.

A broad spectrum of social consequences of conflict can thus be linked to decline in public health. The existing literature on the public health consequences of conflict serves at best to reflect the importance of further exploration of the topic. It asserts that a negative relationship exists between war and public health that goes beyond the direct casualties of war but does not adequately elucidate the causal mechanisms that lead to the indirect effects on health. No comprehensive coherent conceptual framework exists for studying the causes of decline in public health due to conflict, and the empirical work has not been able to explain thoroughly this relationship over time. Some of the questions that the existing literature leaves unanswered pertain to (1) the elements of health achievement, (2) the temporal dynamics of the relationship between conflict and public health, (3) the real means through which conflict affects public health, and (4) the influence of the characteristics of conflict on health.

I present a framework through which the linkages between conflict and public health can be better explained; this framework is illustrated in

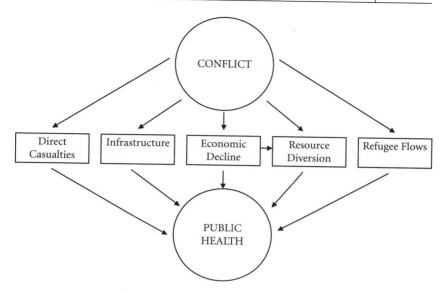

Figure 3.1. Conflict and Health: The Conceptual Framework

Figure 3.1. Conflict has direct and indirect effects on public health. In addition to the direct casualties of war, conflict adversely affects public health through creation of refugee flows and forced migration, economic and social decline, diversion of resources, and damage to the infrastructure.

The Effect of Conflict on Levels of Health Achievement

Conflict can kill and wound the population of a society. Direct casualties of war include the soldiers who lose their lives or are wounded during the fighting. Conflict often results in civilian casualties as well. Civilians die and are wounded in attacks either as collateral damage or as actual targets. Other than the immediate loss of civilian and military life that occurs during conflict, a number of people are left with long-term or lifelong disabilities. Hence, the direct effects of conflict on health are severe and quite obvious. These effects are manifest in the number of battle deaths, the number of people wounded during the conflict, and the number of people disabled as a result of conflict.

The conflict data and literature adequately reveal that conflict kills and wounds people. However, for every direct military death there is at least one civilian death during a conflict, and about a quarter of those killed during war are women (Murray et al. 2002). In the year 2000, conflict-related deaths in the world were estimated at 310,000, more than half of which were in sub-Saharan Africa (Murray et al. 2002). In addition to war mortality, conflict is responsible for significant numbers of nonfatal injuries and disabilities, such as the effect of land mines. Large numbers of military personnel as well as civilians sustain nonfatal injuries during phases of violent conflict that result in subsequent disabilities. I argue that the public health of a society will decline or be negatively influenced by the occurrence of militarized conflict and this effect will vary with the intensity of conflict. Stewart and Fitzgerald (2001) assert that in evaluating the human cost of war, it is essential to take into account "those casualties not directly due to the physical violence, but which result from lack of access to food and health facilities, which can lead to deaths on a massive scale as well as widespread debilitation" (5).

The impact of war on health, however, does not occur in isolation of other relevant social, political, and economic factors. In order to assess health achievement adequately, it is important to take into account the major influences on public health. Wealth, trade, and democracy are among factors that wield significant influence over a society's ability to provide public health. Baum and Lake (2003) argue that democracy has a positive effect on public health, particularly in poorer states. The wealthier a state is, the more resources it has for public health provisions. Trade, as a possible generator of wealth, can also contribute to better public health. Conflict leads to a decline in levels of health achievement, but that effect can best be understood if the relationship between health and its other determinants, such as democracy, is also considered. Moreover, the effect of war on public health levels may be different in the short term and the long run. It can be argued that the effect of war would be more devastating on public health immediately following a conflict, while in the long run, societies are better able to adjust to the shocks brought about by violent conflict.

I hypothesize that the overall level of public health will decline if a state is involved in conflict, and the intensity of the conflict is positively related to the decline in health outcomes. Furthermore, decline in health achievement is likely to be more drastic in the short term after the war but continues in the long run. States with higher levels of wealth and economic openness enjoy higher levels of health outputs, and health achievement is also higher in democratic states. The effect of violent conflict on overall levels of public health—also referred to as health achievement or output—is examined in Chapters 4 and 5.

Type of Conflict

Ghobarah et al. (2003) argue that civil wars are particularly detrimental to public health. The existing literature on conflict and public health focuses on civil wars and argues that the effect of civil wars on public health is higher due to all the fighting and devastation occurring on the soil of the same state. However, interstate wars fought on a belligerent's own soil may have equally devastating effects on the well-being of a society. For example, the 1991 Gulf War had lasting effects on public health in Iraq but did not influence levels of public health in the United States. I explore the effect of both interstate and intrastate conflict on public health and I argue that any kind of violent conflict is likely to lower the level of health outputs in a society. Civil wars may be seen as being more devastating since they are always fought on a state's own territory, but the analyses in this book evaluate the linkages between conflict and public health by examining the effect of both interstate and intrastate conflict on health achievement of states. Thus the empirical models analyzed in the proceeding chapters include both types of conflicts.

Infrastructure

Some of the most intense effects of conflict on public health occur through damage to the infrastructure. Evans et al. (2001) mention that the *World Health Report 2000* defines three main goals of health systems: "improving health, increasing responsiveness to the legitimate demands of the population, and ensuring that financial burdens are distributed fairly" (307). King and Martin (2001) assert that advancements in war technology have resulted in making war more dangerous for civilian populations than for soldiers due to the magnitude of the public health consequences of war, as combatants target the infrastructure of the cities of their opponents, which results in severe public health repercussions for the civilian populations. Damage to both the general infrastructure (such as roads, bridges, and transportation services) and elements of the infrastructure specifically related to health (including hospitals, pharmacies, and medical personnel) can seriously impair a state's ability to offer adequate health care. For instance, destruction of the power grid affects the working of water and sewage pumping stations, giving rise to numerous public health problems. Transportation and communication get disrupted due to destruction of roads, railroads, bridges, and so forth. Consequently, the distribution of food, water, medicine, and relief supplies is interrupted and the availability and mobility of health care providers are adversely affected (Ghobarah et al. 2004). Functioning health care facilities entail working hospitals, access to and availability of physicians and medical staff, and adequate levels of medical supplies. Wars can entirely destroy health care facilities, such as hospitals, or severely limit their capacity to serve the community's health care needs. In addition to possible direct damage to health care facilities, conflict can affect public health through damage to standard determinants of infrastructure.

The negative effect on public health is exacerbated by combatant states' inability to rebuild their infrastructures. Conflict reduces the productivity of the economy and leaves a society with fewer resources. And, given heightened security concerns, some of the available resources tend to get diverted toward military purposes. Public health resources, such as physicians and hospitals, may be mobilized for the war effort and become unavailable to civilians. After the end of a conflict, there is likely to be a diversion of resources from public health to economic recovery. As a result, the rebuilding required to restore provision of public health to previous levels takes a long time; in the meantime, health indicators might continue to decline.

Violent conflict has the effect of concurrently reducing health care capacity through widespread damage to the infrastructure and increasing health care needs among the military and civilian populations. The infrastructure of a state may be directly targeted by enemy forces or be destroyed during attacks on military targets, and the linkages among infrastructure and health care are numerous and salient. The 1991 Gulf War is an excellent illustration of the difficulty in targeting the military machine of a state without causing debilitating damage to the civilian infrastructure. That war also demonstrated the important role that infrastructural destruction can play in the health care capacities of a society. The infrastructure of Baghdad in particular suffered severe damage and, in the absence of viable post-conflict reconstruction, health achievement continued to decline for years after the official cessation of conflict. In Chapter 6, I assess the linkages among conflict, societal infrastructure, and public health achievement. I present the simple argument that conflict negatively affects key elements of the infrastructure of a state and, in addition to the direct effects of conflict on population health, infrastructural damage reduces health outputs.

Diversion of Resources

Governments often have to make difficult decisions regarding the allocation of scarce resources among competing uses, such as expenditures on public health. In fact, in most of the world, maintaining the quality of life that was achieved during the twentieth century has become a challenge due to lack of resources available for public health and disease reduction (Michaud et al. 2001). Simply stated, societies that allocate more resources to health have better public health outputs, and involvement in conflict further complicates the already difficult decisions regarding allocation of resources to public health. During conflict, more resources are allocated to military uses to meet the new security goals of the state, and consequently, fewer resources are available for health expenditures. In fact, involvement in violent conflict could lead to a direct withdrawal of resources from health care to facilitate the needs of the military and other defense expenses. Moreover, the economic consequences of conflict could lead to an overall reduction of wealth in the society as the economic infrastructure deteriorates. This would lead to a decrease in the total resources available in the affected society as well as the need to divert resources from public health spending to military expenditures. Conflict thus results in a smaller pool of resources and fewer of the available resources go toward health spending.

Therefore, the disruption of economic infrastructure that occurs during conflict leads to economic repercussions, including a decline in public expenditures apportioned for health care. The longer a state is involved in a militarized conflict, the worse will be the economic consequences of that conflict. Hence, protracted conflict is likely to lead to an increase in the scarcity of available resources as well as an increase in the diversion of resources to military uses. Collier (1999) argues that war has "large effects on both the level and composition of economic activity" and that war results in economic decline "partly because war directly reduces production and partly because it causes a gradual loss of the capital stock due to destruction, dissaving, and the substitution of portfolios abroad" (181). Prolonged conflict is likely to result in more severe economic repercussions and thus more contraction in resources available for and spent on public health. Although Collier's discussion of the economic consequences of conflict is limited to civil wars, I argue that both intrastate and interstate conflicts adversely affect public health through economic decline and diversion of resources. Poorer economies are particularly vulnerable to the negative effects of "exogenous shocks" that might be caused by conflict, bearing serious consequences for trade flows and domestic markets for labor and credit (Fitzgerald 2001). The microeconomic disequilibria brought about by war influence macroeconomic policy and allocation of resources. Even if social and health spending is maintained at current monetary levels, inflation may decrease the real value of the resources allocated for those purposes. In that case, social spending would actually have to be increased to maintain prewar levels of services.

I argue that involvement in violent conflict causes a reduction in social spending, including public health expenditures, compared to prewar levels of spending. Moreover, states involved in conflict are likely to experience a decline in wealth and rates of economic growth, exacerbating trade-offs in defense and social welfare. Chapter 7 presents empirical analyses of these economic effects.

Forced Migration

Conflict results in forced migration of large groups of people, which can lead to the spread of infectious diseases and epidemics. These flows of people occur under suboptimal health conditions; people are often placed in crowded situations without adequate access to health facilities, medicine, clean water, food, and sanitation. Consequently, it is difficult to contain diseases or provide vaccinations. Merely in the past two decades, "conflicts have collectively been responsible for uprooting over 60 million people—more than the combined populations of 13 Western European countries" (Carballo and Nerukar 2001, 556). Global migration has seen a drastic rise in recent decades due to economic reasons as well as refugee flows. Improvements in communication and transportation have facilitated fast mass movements of refugees, leading to health repercussions for the migrant group as well as the host country.

Accounting for increasing numbers of refugees since the end of World War II, Weiner (1996) finds:

> first, that the increases are largely the result of conflicts within states, primarily, though not exclusively, because of ethnic conflicts, while wars between states remain a significant but diminishing source of refugee flows; second, that the average number of refugees per conflict has been increasing more rapidly than the number of countries producing refugees; and finally, that there are "neighborhoods" or entire regions containing countries with high levels of violence and refugee flow. (6)

Since the end of the Cold War, the bulk of violent conflict in the world has occurred within states. Intrastate conflicts are more likely than interstate war to produce refugees since the warring factions are generally fighting for control over territory in the same state. Increase in control of a region by one group results in displacement of members of the other group in that region. These displaced people either cross national borders to gain refugee status in another state or become internally displaced persons within their own country. Weiss (1999) argues that the nature of intrastate conflict not only gives rise to a generation of displaced people, it also makes it difficult to exercise established principles of humanitarian law. Since the actors involved in civil strife are not state governments, they do not conform to international humanitarian norms. Internal conflicts are marked by "the direct targeting of civilians and relief personnel; the use of foreign aid to fuel conflicts and war economies; and the protracted nature of many so-called emergencies which in fact last for decades" (364). Humanitarian law is often useless in civil wars since the conflict is not controlled by "governments and regular armies whose interests [a]re often served by respecting the rules of warfare" (Weiss 1999, 364). The prevalence of intrastate conflict in the current international system has made refugee flows an important security issue. The main policy question raised by the issue of population displacement due to conflict is how to prevent the conditions within states that lead to the creation of refugees. This would entail prevention of large-scale internal conflict, or tenacious international involvement to ensure that groups within states are not compelled to migrate.

Although a large number of displaced people remain within their own states, my study focuses on the effect of forced migration across countries on public health. Both the migrant group and the population of the host state may experience a deterioration in their well-being as the host society deals with the influx of refugees. The effect of refugee flows on population health is generally felt in the state that receives the refugees, thus demonstrating how the social consequences of conflict can diffuse beyond the states that are actually involved in war. The argument regarding the effect of forced migration on health in Chapter 8 rests on three hypotheses. First, conflict forces groups of people to abandon their homes and enter another state as refugees. Second, refugees are more likely to migrate to states with lower levels of violent conflict due to concerns for their safety. And third, the health achievement of states to which large groups of refugees migrate will decline.

IMPLICATIONS FOR HUMAN SECURITY

Assessing the health consequences of war deepens our comprehension of the costs of war. State leaderships take the expected costs of a war into consideration before making the decision to engage in armed conflict. Higher expected costs of war can play an important role in deterring states and other groups from initiating militarized conflict. It can also influence the response of the side that is being attacked. Since more than half of the deaths due to violent conflict occur among the civilian population, disregarding the effect of war on people would be ignoring one of the most harrowing costs of war. Therefore, an understanding of how violent conflict affects the well-being and health of societies would factor into the decisions of state-level policy makers and possibly serve to prevent conflict. High cost of war in terms of human suffering would reduce the incentives for involvement in conflict and induce policy makers to pursue nonviolent means of con-flict resolution, including various tracks of diplomacy and involvement of international organizations.

Even if the realization of the human costs of war does not prevent con-flict, it would nonetheless influence the manner in which policy makers and practitioners approach health-related consequences of war. An evolution of norms that encourages minimizing the negative effects of war on civilians and a reduction in collateral damage would compel war strategists to devise ways to avoid disrupting the lives of civilian populations. During the 1991 Gulf War, the Iraqi infrastructure, particularly in Baghdad, was destroyed to cripple the Iraqi war machine. Roads, bridges, power plants, and water supplies were disabled to impede the operations of the military. However, that strategy resulted in widespread and lasting misery for the Iraqi people and incapacitated their health care system. Taking the health consequences of war into account would discourage a battle strategy that entails such prodigious repercussions for noncombatants in a population. Hence, fail-ing conflict prevention, an emphasis on the effect of war on people would affect decisions regarding the conduct of war.

Making the health impact of conflict a priority calls for international involvement in situations where domestic or interstate conflict may cause public health issues. International organizations, nongovernmental organi-zations (NGOs), humanitarian aid agencies, and human rights organiza-tions play a significant role in dealing with public health emergencies and the long-term deterioration of health levels caused by violent conflict. A global commitment to preventing, reducing, controlling, and eliminating the health costs of war would lead to active participation of governmental and nongovernmental actors at all levels—from local to global—in dealing with public health challenges.

In furthering the awareness of the human cost of war, the goals of this project are consistent with the goals of the broader ideas regarding human security. This study aims to make the health consequences of conflict a priority in policy making so as to prevent violence at the collective level. The second goal is to make relevant actors understand the importance of minimizing the negative effects of war on health and providing the affected groups with adequate assistance. Third, this study reflects the importance of the involvement of a wide range of actors—from international organizations to individuals—in ensuring that the health effects of conflict are appropriately addressed.

CONCLUSION

Violent conflict negatively affects the health of populations in direct as well as indirect ways. In addition to the immediate death and injury caused by war, there are continuing effects that lead to a decline in public health in the short, medium, and long term. The immediate and short-term effects of conflict on health are reflected in declines in overall levels of public health indicators. These effects, however, occur within the political and economic environment of particular states. The extent to which the level of public health decreases due to conflict is also related to factors such as the nature of a state's political institutions and its economic might. In the medium to long run, conflict affects the health and well-being of a society through creation of refugee flows, economic decline, resource allocation choices, and general social decline. In the next chapter, I empirically evaluate the effect of conflict on overall levels of population health, using a summary measure of health, in light of relevant political and economic factors.

4

CONFLICT AND LEVELS
OF HEALTH ACHIEVEMENT

IN THE PREVIOUS CHAPTER, I outlined some important elements of the relationship between conflict and public health and the ways in which war can lead to a decline in levels of health. The consequences of violent conflict permeate countless aspects of a society and are not limited to the political and economic institutions of a state. In this chapter, I examine the effect of militarized conflict on the populations of states by evaluating the relationship between war and public health, taking into account relevant political and economic factors, such as democracy and wealth. I assess the effect of war on overall levels of health achievement in states, as indicated by a summary measure of public health. To examine the relationship between violent conflict and health, I test the following hypotheses: (1) the overall level of public health will decline if a state is involved in conflict, and the intensity of the conflict is positively related to the decline in health outcomes; (2) the decline in health achievement is likely to be greater in the short term after the war, but overall levels of health outputs continue to be affected in the long run; (3) states with higher levels of wealth and economic openness enjoy higher levels of health outputs; and (4) higher levels of democracy are associated with higher levels of health outcomes.[3]

I argue that interstate and intrastate conflicts negatively influence the health achievement of states and, therefore, the well-being of their populations. I assess the magnitude of this relationship by analyzing data on aggregate levels of public health in all states between 1999 and 2002 in light of relevant political and economic factors, including wealth, trade, and regime type. Involvement in violent conflict lowers the overall levels of public health, especially in countries without established democratic institutions and with lower levels of income; there is a decline in health achievement in the short term and the long run. The findings suggest that the negative effect of war on health is closely linked to the levels of income, trade, and democracy.

MEASURING PUBLIC HEALTH

Most studies of population health use summary measures of public health that combine information on mortality and nonfatal health outcomes to express the health of a population as a single number and include inputs such as age-specific mortality and the epidemiology of nonfatal health outcomes. Such summary measures are useful for comparing the health of populations across states and time. One of the summary measures of public health used in recent literature is Health-Adjusted Life Expectancy (HALE), provided by the World Health Organization (WHO). HALE was previously referred to as Disability-Adjusted Life Expectancy (DALE). The HALE measure subtracts the number of years an individual is expected to spend with a disability as a burden of disease from the total life expectancy at birth. Another measure, derived from HALE, aggregates data on health outcomes by gender and five age groups and is referred to as Disability-Adjusted Life Years (DALY). Ghobarah et al. (2003) use this measure as the dependent variable in their study of conflict and health. Although DALYs provide information about life expectancy in certain population groups and deaths resulting from particular diseases, this measure is only available for 1999. The analyses in this chapter use HALE as the summary measure of public health due to its availability for a longer period of time. Moreover, for the purposes of this analysis, the population and disease groupings are not necessary since the goal of this chapter is to gauge the impact of war on the overall levels of health. Thus the added advantage of data availability for multiple years is more important. Disaggregated measures of public health, for longer periods of time, are assessed in Chapter 5.

Accounting for Disability: Health-Adjusted Life Expectancy (HALE)

To test the hypotheses posited in this study, I examine aggregate public health levels in all member states of the World Health Organization from 1999 to 2002. To assess the effect of war on health, I also analyze changes in HALE by comparing the figures for the current and previous years.

The HALE measure is estimated by the Burden of Disease project of the World Health Organization, employing a methodology that links incidence and causes of disease to information on "both short-term and long-term health outcomes, including impairments, functional limitations (disability), restrictions in participation in usual roles (handicap), and death" (Mathers et al. 2000, 1). The measure expresses the number of years that individuals in a population are expected to live in "full health," excluding time spent in states lower than ideal health as described by an accepted norm for a population. One advantage of using HALE as an expression of levels of health is the ease with which the notion of "healthy life" can be comprehended by audiences who are not well-versed in more technical health measures. HALE is an accessible measure because health is expressed as a single number, made even more intuitive by using years of life as the unit of expression. The accessibility of this measure to a wide variety of disciplines as well as policy makers makes it highly attractive and valuable. Mathers et al. (2001a) describe HALE as the best Summary Measure of Public Health (SMPH) to reflect the overall level of health in a population.

Figure 4.1 illustrates the differences in the total life expectancies and HALEs in Jamaica and Venezuela. The two countries have practically identical life expectancies, approximately 73 years. However, the HALE in Jamaica is about seven years longer than in Venezuela. This indicates that although people in both populations tend to live the same average number of years, a member of the Jamaican population is expected to spend about 68 years in full health, while people in Venezuela live only 61 years without disease or disability. This measure, thus, captures quality of life in addition to life

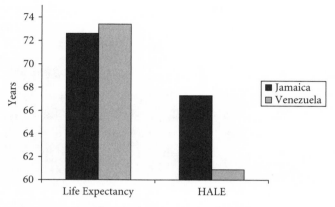

Figure 4.1. HALE and Total Life Expectancy in Two Countries

expectancy. HALE is lower than simple life expectancy in all states, but the degree of this difference varies across countries and reflects the prevalence of suboptimal health conditions in that society.

Estimating HALE

Health expectancy is the term used for summary measures of population health that estimate the expectation of years of life lived in various health states. Figure 4.2 shows HALE for 191 countries from 1999 to 2002. The simplest way to calculate health expectancy is to use data from self-reported health surveys that attempt to determine the health of individuals at various levels of severity. This approach has been quite useful in some states, such as Australia and Canada. However, the use of self-reported surveys for compiling data to calculate summary measures of health raises the issue of comparability across populations and time due to variations in data collection methods and the quality of the data. Moreover, it is not easy to assign weights to specific health conditions to be able to discern the extent to which various conditions affect the health of people. To address this issue, the HALE measurement includes analyses of epidemiological information on specific health conditions. The WHO's *World Health Report 2002* describes the methods used in calculating HALE:

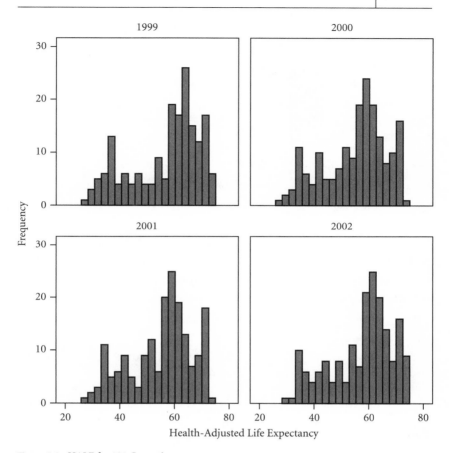

Figure 4.2. HALE for 191 Countries

Analyses of over 50 national health surveys for the calculation of healthy life expectancy in the *World Health Report 2000* identified severe limitations in the comparability of self-reported health status data from different populations, even when identical survey instruments and methods are used. The WHO Household Survey Study carried out 69 representative household surveys in 60 Member States in 2000 and 2001 using a new health status instrument based on the International Classification of Functioning, Disability and Health, which seeks information from a representative sample of respondents on their current states of health according to six core domains. These domains were identified from an extensive review of the currently available health status measurement instruments. To overcome the problem of comparability of self-reported health data, the WHO survey instrument used performance tests and vignettes to calibrate self-reported health on selected domains such as cognition, mobility and vision. WHO has developed several statistical methods for correcting biases in self-reported health using these data, based on the hierarchical ordered probit (HOPIT) model. The calibrated responses are used to estimate the true prevalence of different states of health by age and sex. (World Health Organization 2002b, 172–173)[4]

The first step in these calculations is to develop weighted disability prevalence estimates based on age and sex for each country, using epidemiological information on specific conditions. The second step is the "construction of latent health factor scores from representative population health surveys" (Mathers et al. 2000, 13). The next step is to estimate weighted disability prevalence from the scores derived from self-reported surveys in a way so as to maximize comparability by adjusting for self-report biases. Finally, these disability estimates and life expectancy measures are used to calculate HALE, combining survey data and epidemiological analyses. These calculations are conducted through "Sullivan's method," which involves using the "observed prevalence of disability at each age in the current population at a given point of time to divide the hypothetical years of life lived by a period life table cohort at different ages into years with and without disability" (Mathers et al. 2001b, 122). Appendix B illustrates the calculation of HALE through "Sullivan's method."

The HALE measure is available for all WHO member states for the years 1999 through 2002 (see Appendix C). This is the most appropriate single-number indicator of overall health levels due to the comprehensive nature of the data and the careful calculations it employs. This measure provides an efficient way to compare health outputs across populations and years.

INFLUENCES ON HEALTH OUTCOMES

As discussed in Chapter 3, violent conflict may affect public health through a host of means, including damage to the infrastructure of the society, interruptions in access to basic services such as water and transportation, lack of availability of health care personnel, and diversion of economic resources from public health to military uses. Other indirect effects of conflict on health include food shortages, famine, and economic decline.

One important factor in determining health achievement is the nature of political institutions that govern a state. Democratic states are more likely to be sensitive to the health care needs of their populations since the population possesses channels to voice their grievances, as well as the ability not to reelect the incumbent leadership. The extent to which health achievement declines in the wake of conflict, however, is also related to the level of wealth in the affected society. Broadly speaking, wealthier societies are better able to maintain higher levels of public health. I argue that the higher the level of a state's income, the higher the overall level of health. Similarly, since trade serves as a means to generate revenue, states with high levels of trade will also experience better health care in general as well as during times of conflict. This suggests a positive relationship between economic openness and provision of public health.

I hypothesize, first, that involvement in conflict lowers the overall levels of public health in states. Second, I expect a positive relationship between democracy and levels of health outputs. Third, I argue that populations of states with higher levels of income and trade openness enjoy better health provisions. I also control for population size in my models.

Conflict

Involvement in violent conflict negatively affects the health achievement of a state due to the direct effects of war in terms of military and civilian casualties. The magnitude of the health impact of wars varies immensely, but it is rare for a war—interstate or intrastate—to incur no costs in terms of human well-being. For example, according to the United Kingdom's Department for International Development, the war in Bosnia caused serious repercussions for the Bosnian population:

> The civil war was disastrous, the toll on the country and its citizens a catalogue of misery. It left an estimated 250,000 people dead, 240,000 wounded, and 25,000 permanently disabled. Some 50,000 children were wounded. About 50,000 people still require rehabilitation and 15 percent of the population suffer from post traumatic

stress disorder. There are estimated 800,000 externally displaced people still refugees abroad. In addition there are about 1 million internally displaced people, living within BH, but not in their home communities. (United Kingdom Department of International Development 2003)

The Liberian crisis has caused the spread of diseases such as cholera and diarrhea due to lack of clean drinking water and widespread malnutrition. Although some of the hospitals continue to function in Monrovia, the chaotic conditions of the city make it impossible for most people to reach the hospitals. Moreover, medical supplies are scarce because of transportation issues: "Due to the ongoing fighting in Monrovia, vaccines estimated at USD 250,000 stored in National Drugs Services (NDS) are at risk to be lost for lack of fuel. The port where fuel is available is controlled by the LURD group and not accessible from Central Monrovia" (World Health Organization 2003).

The first independent variable in this study is *Conflict*. Health achievement is likely to decline during and after a conflict due to the direct and indirect ways in which violent conflict affects the health of populations. Ghobarah et al. (2003, 2004) operationalize civil wars as the number of civil war deaths, which raises the issue of endogeneity since the HALE measure incorporates life expectancy and deaths. My conflict variables, on the other hand, measure both the presence of conflict at various levels of intensity and the frequency of conflict. Moreover, I include both civil and interstate conflict. To assess the presence of conflict, I consult data from the Peace Research Institute of Oslo (PRIO) Dataset on Armed Conflict (Gleditsch et al. 2002). These data measure conflict according to both its intensity and its type, including domestic and international conflict. Following the PRIO guidelines, I categorize conflict as *major conflict* and *minor conflict*. Major conflict refers to militarized conflicts that result in at least 1,000 battle deaths in a given year; minor conflict refers to conflicts in which there have been at least 25 deaths in a given year and more than 1,000 deaths in the history of the conflict. I also include a variable for the number of conflicts in which a state was involved in a given year, thus assessing separately the effects of the intensity and frequency of conflict. It should be noted that most of the

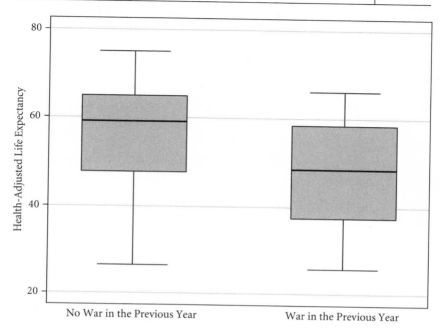

Figure 4.3. War and HALE

conflicts during the period examined were internal conflicts or civil wars. In general, I expect violent conflict to have a negative effect on public health, as measured by HALE. An examination of the bivariate relationship between conflict and HALE reveals a substantial decline in health both due to the presence of conflict and with an increase in the number of conflicts in which a state is involved. Figure 4.3 is a box plot of HALE for countries that did or did not experience a war in the previous year during the period studied in this analysis; it shows that HALE levels are clearly lower in the presence of a war. About eight years of healthy life are lost in countries that were involved in a war in the previous year. Similarly, Figure 4.4 considers the number of conflicts in which a state was involved in the previous year and reveals a monotonically declining pattern in median HALE; as frequency of conflict increases, HALE decreases.

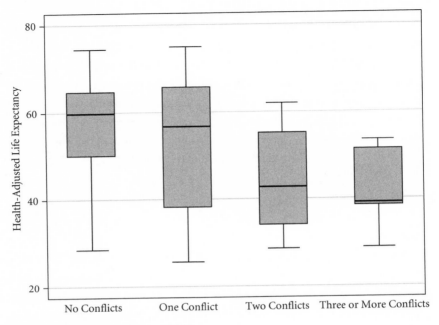

Figure 4.4. Conflict Frequency and HALE

Democracy

I expect to find higher levels of health achievement in states that possess highly democratic regimes. It is widely accepted that democratic regimes are more responsive to the needs of their populations, including those that are health-related. The perpetuation of the leadership is closely related to the well-being of the public in democratic systems, which suggests that democratic governments would be more likely to allocate greater resources to the public health infrastructure. Ghobarah et al. (2004) find that democracies allocate more public spending to health care than nondemocracies; they do not, however, evaluate the direct effect of democracy on health. Interestingly, many highly autocratic societies enjoy levels of public health that are very close to industrialized democracies of Western Europe and North America. For instance, in the years 1999 to 2001, Cuba, Qatar, and Saudi Arabia had average health achievement scores of 67.2, 61.97, and 61.43, respectively. These states supported some of the most autocratic regimes in the international system, according to the *POLITY IV* democracy scores for these years. The health achievement levels in Norway, the United Kingdom, and the United States were 71.07, 70.17, and 68.33, respectively. Unlike the first set of countries, these states maintained the highest possible democracy score (10 on the POLITY scale). The differences in the health outcomes of these groups of highly autocratic and highly democratic states are by no means as great as one would expect if a linear relationship existed between democracy and health outcomes. On the other hand, public health scores in Zambia, Liberia, and the Democratic Republic of the Congo—as measured by HALE—range from 30 to 37, significantly lower than the autocratic and the democratic regimes mentioned earlier. The *POLITY Scores* of this last group of countries were between −1 and 1 during the years being examined. These states, therefore, were neither completely autocratic nor highly democratic.

This hints at a curvilinear relationship between the regime type of a state and the level of public health. But I argue that such a curvilinear effect would exist only in the absence of the variable for wealth. The highly autocratic states that maintain high levels of health outputs also enjoy per-capita GDPs close to the wealthiest Western democracies, which might explain the weakly curvilinear bivariate relationship between democracy and healthy life expectancy revealed in Figure 4.5. Accordingly, I suggest that it is proliferation of wealth in society rather than the policies of the regime that accounts for better public health. Democracies, on the other hand, are conscientious about their public health provisions due to the norms and values embedded in their institutional structures and the ability of the population to oust the incumbent regime in the next election. Governments often have to make difficult decisions regarding the allocation of scarce resources among competing uses, such as expenditures on public health (Russett 1969; Mintz 1989), and conflict further complicates these decisions by increasing the security needs of the state. The governmental systems in democratic states are more likely to prioritize in favor of health expenditures than those of autocratic regimes. The latter are not accountable to their populations for their resource allocation decisions and are more likely to divert resources toward military expenditures to enhance their power. Therefore, I argue that levels of democracy are positively related to public health.

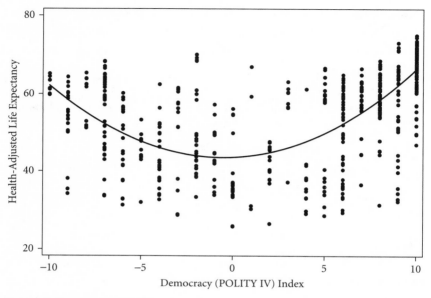

Figure 4.5. Democracy and HALE

I hypothesize that the level of *Democracy* in a state will have a positive effect on the well-being of a society. States that are highly democratic experience higher levels of health achievement than those with autocratic regimes or lower levels of democracy. To measure the level of democracy, I use the *POLITY IV scores*. These scores range from −10 to 10, with higher scores denoting higher levels of democracy. Thus, a state with a score of 10 is considered completely democratic, and one with a score of −10 is an autocracy. This is a widely accepted indicator of regime type and is employed extensively in quantitative analyses of international relations. The POLITY IV dataset provides the regime type for all independent states in the international system, with a total population of at least 500,000 in a given year, for the period from 1800 to 2007. For the purposes of compiling these democracy scores,

> democracy is conceived as three essential, interdependent elements. One is the presence of institutions and procedures through which citizens can express effective preferences about alternative policies and leaders. Second is the existence of

institutionalized constraints on the exercise of power by the executive. Third is the guarantee of civil liberties to all citizens in their daily lives and in acts of political participation. (Marshall and Jaggers 2009, 13)

Therefore, the democracy score for each state is obtained from codings of the openness and competitiveness of executive recruitment, competitiveness of political participation, and constraints on the power of the chief executive (Marshall and Jaggers 2009). The *POLITY scores* thus offer a quantitative measure of regime type based on universally agreed-upon elements of democratic principles. Moreover, the temporal and spatial breadth of the dataset makes it ideal for empirical analyses that require an indicator for regime type. In the analyses in this chapter, a squared term for *POLITY scores* is also included to test for a possible curvilinear relationship between the covariates and the dependent variable.

Economic Factors

It is generally accepted that poverty and disease are closely related and that poorer states do not enjoy the same levels of health as richer states. Inequality in health achievement across states is a major concern for scholars of development (Leon and Walt 2001; Sen 2001; Zwi 2001). At higher levels of wealth, states are able to provide better preventive and curative health care. Leon and Walt (2001), however, warn against ignoring the effect of higher levels of health on the economic well-being of states:

> In much of what is written about the link between health and wealth, it is often implicitly assumed that the direction of causality is from wealth (or poverty) to health (or disease). However, the possibility that either at the individual or population level, there can be a causal link running from health to wealth needs to be considered. (5)

A healthier population is more productive and contributes to economic activity more than an ailing population. Nonetheless, economic resources are necessary for the provision of health care and the effect of wealth on health is potent in the short run and in the long term. I argue that levels of wealth are positively related to health achievement, with the causal arrow

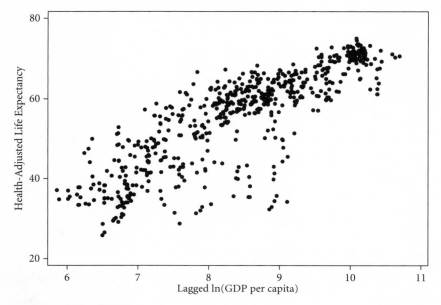

Figure 4.6. GDP and HALE

running from wealth to health. Figure 4.6 shows a positive relationship between national income and HALE in a bivariate context for the time period under consideration.

Trade openness is associated with economic prosperity, and it may be argued that states with higher levels of trade are likely to enjoy higher standards of health achievement. In the current international atmosphere of globalization and interdependence, open economies fare better than closed economies and are able to provide higher standards of public services, including health care. Trade acts as an economic stimulus and has a similar effect on health outputs as GDP. Therefore, I expect trade openness to have a positive effect on health achievement.

The covariates in this analysis include *Per-Capita GDP* (gross domestic product), *Trade Openness*, and *Population*. Data on wealth and economic openness were obtained from the Penn World Table (Heston et al. 2002, 2006). The income or wealth of states is measured by per-capita GDP expressed in constant prices and in U.S. dollars. Trade openness is measured

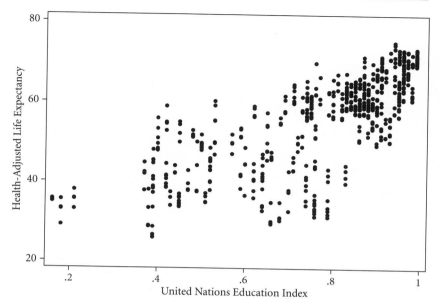

Figure 4.7. Education and HALE

by the total volume of exports and imports as a proportion of GDP. The larger this percentage, the more open the economy, since a larger proportion of its income is being generated through trade with other states. Population statistics come from the World Bank's World Development Index and are expressed in millions. I also control for education; the level of *Education* of a population is measured by an education index used in the United Nations Human Development Index; see Figure 4.7 for the relationship between education and HALE. This education index is based on the adult literacy rate and the combined gross enrollment ratio for primary, secondary, and tertiary schools (United Nations Development Programme 2004).[5]

I argue that both wealth and openness have a positive effect on public health, and I include a variable that measures the interaction effect between wealth and openness to evaluate whether the influence of openness is different in wealthy versus poor states. Taking into account the wealth— or poverty—of states when examining the effect of economic openness on health will address speculation about the benefits of globalization for

Table 4.1. Summary Statistics: Levels and Long-Term Effects

Variables	Mean	Standard Deviation	Minimum	Maximum
Dependent Variable				
HALE	55.64	12.03	25.8	75
Independent Variables				
Lagged Major Conflict	0.06	0.23	0	1
Lagged Minor Conflict	0.07	0.25	0	1
Lagged Conflict (count)	0.31	0.72	0	6
Lagged POLITY score	3.52	6.36	−10	10
Lagged POLITY score squared	52.75	34.65	0	100
Lagged ln(Per-Capita GDP)	8.43	1.14	5.85	10.44
Lagged ln(Trade Openness)	4.28	0.54	2.54	6.09
Lagged ln(Population)	9.20	1.50	6.06	14.06
Education	0.77	0.20	0.16	0.99

NOTE: $N = 548$.

Table 4.2. Summary Statistics: Changes and Short-Term Effects

Variables	Mean	Standard Deviation	Minimum	Maximum
Dependent Variable				
ΔHALE	0.36	2.4	−12	7.8
Independent Variables				
Major Conflict	0.05	0.21	0	1
Minor Conflict	0.07	0.26	0	1
Conflict (count)	0.28	0.66	0	6
Lagged ΔPOLITY score	0.12	1.16	−12	10
Lagged ΔPOLITY score squared	1.36	9.86	0	144
Lagged Δln(Per-Capita GDP)	0.04	0.13	−0.91	0.92
Lagged Δln(Trade Openness)	0.02	0.17	−0.72	0.69
Lagged Δln(Population)	0.02	0.06	−0.15	0.98

NOTE: $N = 413$.

lesser-developed states. Education is expected to be positively related to health, since educated populations are better capable of making decisions, such as taking advantage of public health programs, that would contribute to higher health levels (Ghobarah et al. 2004). The summary statistics for all of the variables included in the analyses are presented in Tables 4.1 and 4.2.

ANALYSIS AND RESULTS

The fact that these data comprise repeated observations on a large number of cross-sectional units raises the specter of both temporal correlation and nonconstant error variance. To address these issues, I adopt the method of generalized estimating equations (GEE) (Liang and Zeger 1986; Zorn 2001). This approach has been shown to provide consistent and asymptotically efficient estimates of the parameters of interest. In particular, I estimate GEE models with a first-order autoregressive temporal covariance structure.

I estimate two models to test my hypotheses. The first model measures the effect of the independent variables on the overall level of public health as expressed by HALE for a given year ($Y_{it} = X_{it}\beta + \mu_{it}$). The second model employs the change in public health, taking the difference between HALE for the current year and the previous year ($\Delta Y_{it} = \Delta X_{it}\beta + \epsilon_{it}$). This model assesses the immediate to short-term effect of conflict on health. In order to evaluate adequately the relationship between war and health, it is important to examine both the level of health outputs and the change in health outputs. The effect on the level of health in the first model is a better indicator of how the state would maintain its public health in the long run after the conflict; the change in health achievement due to conflict indicates the direct effect of conflict on health in the year following the violence. For each model, I present separate results for the intensity and the count of conflicts. The variables for the intensity of conflict and the number of conflicts in which a state was involved during the year are not included in the same equation because of multicollinearity.[6]

All independent variables (except *Education*) in the first model have been lagged to take into account the delayed effect of the levels of covariates on HALE. As levels of factors such as GDP and democracy increase or decrease for a given country, effects on health outcomes as measured by HALE take some time to materialize. Lagged independent variables capture temporal effects and, therefore, more adequately reflect the relationship between the covariates and the dependent variable. Moreover, the variables of national income, trade, and population have been logged due to diminishing marginal returns. For instance, if a country's per-capita GDP increases from $100 to $200, the marginal effect on public health would be

Table 4.3. Determinants of Public Health: Levels and Long-Term Effects, 1999–2002

Variables	Intensity	Count
(Constant)	−64.04	−63.68
	(15.05)	(14.72)
Lagged Major Conflict	−1.02	—
	(0.98)	
Lagged Minor Conflict	−0.25	—
	(0.82)	
Lagged Conflict (count)	—	−0.43*
		(0.24)
Lagged POLITY score	0.07	0.08
	(0.08)	(0.09)
Lagged POLITY score squared	0.01	0.01
	(0.01)	(0.01)
Lagged ln(Per-Capita GDP)	10.16**	10.12**
	(2.0)	(1.91)
Lagged ln(Trade Openness)	11.60**	11.34**
	(3.17)	(3.11)
Lagged ln(GDP) × Lagged ln(Openness)	−1.19**	−1.17**
	(0.38)	(0.38)
Lagged ln(Population)	1.22**	1.27**
	(0.34)	(0.33)
Education	21.30**	20.97**
	(3.23)	(3.25)
Wald test	895.58	773.57
(p-value)	(< 0.001)	(< 0.001)
N	548	548

NOTE: Cell entries are coefficient estimates; numbers in parentheses are robust standard errors, clustered by nation. * = $p < .05$; ** = $p < .01$ (one-tailed).

much greater than if a country's per-capita GDP increases from $3,000 to $3,100. Taking the log of the figures for these variables takes into account this issue of diminishing marginal returns and offers more interpretable results. Below I discuss the findings of the two models.

Levels of Health Achievement

The effects of conflict and the other covariates on the level of health achievement are shown in Table 4.3. This model assesses the overall levels of HALE and is a reflection on health output trends in the long run. I find in this model that the overall level of health declines due to involvement in war, but only the coefficient for the number of conflicts is significant. Thus, although the mere presence of conflict may not significantly affect overall long-term levels of public health, as the number of conflicts in which

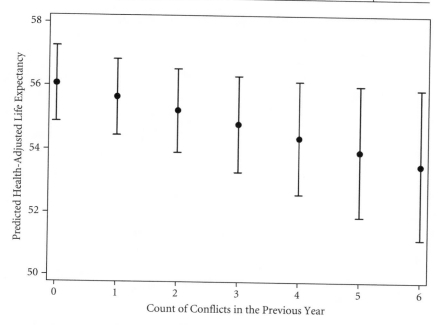

Figure 4.8. The Effect of Conflict on Levels of HALE

states are involved increases, the level of health decreases.[7] This finding, illustrated in Figure 4.8, reveals that every additional (lagged) conflict takes about five months off a nation's health-adjusted life expectancy. This is consistent with the earlier discussion regarding the impact of violent conflict on public health through factors such as destruction of infrastructure, generation of refugee flows, economic decline, and diversion of resources away from health expenditure.[8] These factors reduce the ability of a state to provide public health at a time when the health needs of the population have escalated in the aftermath of militarized conflict. Thus, violent conflict does not just impact the populations of states through creating casualties of war; it also reduces the capability of states to provide adequate health care and public health.

Contrary to expectation, the level of democracy does not have a significantly positive effect on the long-term level of health. As expected, however, there is no evidence of a curvilinear relationship between democracy and health that would suggest that autocracies also enjoy higher levels of health outcomes. It is interesting to note, however, that in a bivariate analysis of the relationship between democracy and health, a curvilinear relationship does exist, but this effect disappears once the model controls for wealth. This explains why some highly repressive but wealthy states, such as Qatar and Saudi Arabia, maintain high levels of public health. The positive effect of democracy on health is also insignificant when looking at the change in HALE.[9] Population size is positively related to health outcomes. The education level of a population has a highly positive effect on health achievement, which supports the expectation that educated populations are better able to maintain higher levels of health due to the ability to make informed choices about health care.

As hypothesized, wealth has a positive effect on levels of health; the higher the GDP of a state, the higher will be the level of its public health. Clearly, wealthier states have the resources to perpetuate better public health systems and maintain higher levels of health outputs. A similar effect exists for trade openness. Open economies have an additional source of income through trade and thus more means for better health provisions. However, when the effects of wealth and openness are interacted, there is a positive effect of openness on health only in poor states; there is no real effect on health in wealthy states. This suggests that overall levels of health outcomes over the long run benefit more significantly from trade openness in poor states than in wealthy states.

Changes in Health Achievement

The second model assesses the changes in the independent variables and HALE, thus giving an indication of the short-term relationships between the explanatory factors and health achievement. The changes in HALE are calculated by taking the difference in the values of HALE for the current and the previous year. Similar calculations are made on the covariates to measure yearly changes. As in the previous model, which assesses the levels of health-adjusted life expectancy, conflict is measured along the dimensions of intensity and count.

The results for this model are shown in Table 4.4, revealing a significant decline in health due to war. This suggests that when a country is involved

Table 4.4. Determinants of Public Health: Changes and Short-Term Effects, 1999–2002

Variables	Intensity	Count
(Constant)	0.13	0.08
	(0.13)	(0.14)
Major Conflict	−1.36**	—
	(0.37)	
Minor Conflict	−0.23	—
	(0.45)	
Conflict (count)	—	0.01
		(0.13)
Lagged ΔPOLITY score	−0.14	−0.11
	(0.10)	(0.10)
Lagged ΔPOLITY score squared	0.02	0.01
	(0.01)	(0.01)
Lagged Δln(Per-Capita GDP)	8.06*	7.22*
	(3.60)	(3.63)
Lagged Δln(Trade Openness)	10.03*	8.49*
	(5.07)	(5.11)
Lagged Δln(GDP) × Lagged Δln(Openness)	−0.99	−0.81
	(0.63)	(0.63)
Lagged Δln(Population)	4.99*	5.19*
	(2.12)	(2.17)
Wald test	35.86	21.90
(p-value)	(< 0.001)	(< 0.005)
N	412	412

NOTE: Cell entries are coefficient estimates; numbers in parentheses are robust standard errors, clustered by nation. * = $p < .05$; ** = $p < .01$ (one-tailed).

in a war, its health achievement is likely to go down in the next year or the short term. This is particularly significant when states are involved in higher-intensity conflicts. Clearly, all the direct effects of war—including combat casualties—are going to take their toll on a society within the short term. The immediate devastation caused by war cannot be compensated in the short term through international assistance and post-conflict reconstruction. In the long run, states recover from the impact of conflict through internal efforts, economic improvement, and external help from other states as well as international organizations. Although nongovernmental organizations—such as Doctors Without Borders (MSF)—have been commendable in entering conflict-ridden areas to provide essential medical care (Taipale 2002), there can be a considerable lag between the onset of conflict and an inflow of international humanitarian and medical assistance.

Intervention by the United Nations and other international organizations has been instrumental in post-conflict social and political recovery in states such as Mozambique (see Russett and Oneal 2001). However, international intervention and peacekeeping often occurs after cease-fires or peace agreements have been established and the warring parties are amenable to an international presence (Goulding 1993). International intervention can help ameliorate the health impact of violent conflict, but such intervention is unlikely to be effective immediately following a conflict. Consequently, the effects of war on population health are felt most drastically in the short term after conflict begins. Not surprisingly, levels of democracy do not have a significant effect on changes in health outcomes immediately after a war.

As in the model looking at levels of health, both national income and economic openness are positively related to health outcomes. However, the interaction of national income and trade openness does not reveal a significant effect in this model. In the model evaluating overall levels of health outputs, both wealth and openness were positively related to public health, but the positive effect of openness on health was limited to poor states. Openness was not positively related to health in wealthier states, suggesting that higher income levels, even in the absence of economic openness, lead to better health achievement. The short-term model, however, does not demonstrate these effects. This implies that free trade does not differentially affect the standard of public health in the short term across wealthy and poor states; the effect of openness is uniformly positive. Education is positively related to health even in the short term. These findings, therefore, demonstrate that the negative effects of conflict on public health can best be explained by taking into account economic and political influences as well as characteristics of states. Levels of wealth, education, and population are positively related to health achievement. Trade openness generally has a positive effect on public health, but to a much greater extent in wealthier states than in poorer countries.

CONCLUSION

The findings of the analyses in this chapter suggest that conflict can undermine health, demonstrate that a number of political and economic factors are important in assessing the effect of conflict on health, and show how the influence of these factors varies across countries with differing characteristics. For instance, the health outcomes of states vary at different levels of wealth, trade, and democracy; the effect of economic openness on health achievement is different for wealthier and poorer states, and these effects further vary in the short term and the long run. Taking temporal dynamics and state characteristics into account contributes to a nuanced understanding of the determinants of health outcomes, reflecting the need for different approaches to health challenges in different parts of the world.

Work on consequences of conflict has mainly focused on states and institutions, including the political, economic, and environmental effects of violence. However, it is more important to study the effect of conflict on the quality of life of states' populations. One of the most significant factors in one's personal well-being is health; similarly, public health reflects the quality of life and well-being of a society. The real costs of violent conflict cannot be understood completely without a clearer comprehension of the mechanisms through which war affects the individuals in a society. There are always normative concerns surrounding war and the use of force, and rhetoric based on these concerns is often used in decisions to avoid violent conflict or to intervene in wars. Empirical evaluation of the effect of war on public health allows us to assess systematically the negative influences of war and enables us to support our normative concerns with empirical evidence. In illuminating the human cost of war, this line of research offers significant implications for the expected utility of violent conflict and provides incentives for conflict prevention. Policy makers invariably take into account the monetary costs of war before becoming involved in a conflict; understanding how state populations are affected by war gives them the opportunity to factor in the cost of war in terms of human security in addition to economic resources and national security.

However, for a more complete understanding of the effect of conflict on health, a time period longer than four years must be studied. Unfortunately, due to the complex nature of the data required for calculating HALE, this measure is only available from 1999 to 2002. HALE was chosen as the dependent variable for this study as it is the best measure that summarizes health as a single number for each country year. Analysis of a longer period of time could evaluate aspects of the relationship between war and health that have not been addressed here due to limitations in data availability. In the next chapter, I assess the effect of conflict on population health over a four-decade period, employing disaggregated measures of public health.

5

A DISAGGREGATED ANALYSIS OF THE IMPACT OF WAR ON HEALTH

IN CHAPTER 4, I examined the relationship between war and overall levels of health achievement, controlling for relevant political and economic factors. In that analysis, national health outputs were measured by the summary measure of public health referred to as Health-Adjusted Life Expectancy (HALE). This measure incorporates a number of aspects of public health, including fatal and nonfatal health outcomes, to express the health of a population as a single figure that indicates the number of years people are likely to spend in the state of "full health." Thus this measure is more useful than simple life expectancy at birth because it reflects life years spent without disease or disability, employs a variety of health conditions in its calculation, facilitates comparisons of health achievement across time and countries, and provides clear and easily interpretable statistical results.

HALE, therefore, may be seen as the single best indicator of population health. However, the data needed for the calculation of HALE have only been collected by the World Health Organization since 1999, limiting the analysis in the previous chapter to four years. In this chapter, I extend the analysis temporally over the past four decades, using disaggregated measures of public health. I examine the effect of the presence and duration of conflict on fertility rates, infant mortality rates, and male and female life expectancies between 1960 and 1999; I also assess the regional differences in these relationships. I maintain that health-adjusted life expectancy better reflects the overall health of a population than disaggregated measures of public health, particularly due to the superior quality of the data used for computing HALE. These disaggregated measures, however, allow for an analysis of the war and health relationship over a much longer period of time.

I hypothesize that public health, as measured by the dependent variables in the analyses in this chapter, deteriorates due to the incidence and protraction of violent conflict. Specifically, I argue that fertility rates and infant mortality rates are likely to increase due to conflict, and male as well as female life expectancies are likely to decrease as a result of war. All of these effects are greater for conflicts of longer duration. Moreover, higher levels of democracy, national income, trade openness—as well as larger populations—are associated with higher levels of health, as manifested by lower fertility and infant mortality rates and higher life expectancy for men and women. I test these hypotheses using measures of public health and data on political and economic factors for all countries from 1960 to 1999. I also expect there to be regional differences among these relationships. In the next section, I outline the independent variables, and then analyze the effect of these covariates on the selected measures of health.

INFLUENCES ON PUBLIC HEALTH

The presence and persistence of violent conflict—whether civil wars or interstate conflict—negatively affect the health and well-being of societies. As discussed in the previous chapter, war has a negative impact on the health of a society through its direct and indirect effects. Direct casualties of war include the soldiers who are killed or wounded during combat and the civilians who are hurt as deliberate targets or collateral damage. But the health of a society is also affected by war through its indirect effects on major components of public health, including destruction of infrastructure and generation of refugee flows (Pedersen 2002; Levy and Sidel 2002). The detrimental effects of war on health may be significantly more severe during civil wars since all the fighting occurs on the soil of a single state (Ghobarah et al. 2003), which is particularly relevant to the current international system since most conflicts in the past two decades have been intrastate wars. Countries with civil wars—such as the Sudan, Liberia, and Sierra Leone—have suffered serious health effects due to the fighting as well as indirect effects of conflict.

The main independent variable in the analyses in this chapter is *Conflict*. I take into account the presence of minor and major conflict as well as the duration of conflict. I expect both the presence and duration of conflict to be negatively related to male and female life expectancies and to be positively related to fertility and infant mortality rates. As in the previous chapter, I consult data from the Peace Research Institute of Oslo (PRIO) on armed conflict (Gleditsch et al. 2002) and I categorize conflict as *Major Conflict* and *Minor Conflict*. *Major Conflict* refers to all militarized conflicts that result in at least 1,000 battle deaths in a given year; *Major Conflict Duration* measures the duration of a conflict. *Minor Conflict* refers to conflicts in which there have been at least 25 deaths in a given year and more than 1,000 deaths in the history of the conflict. *Minor Conflict Duration* is the duration of a minor conflict.

In addition to conflict, important political and economic factors also influence the health outcomes of states. I expect states with higher levels of democracy to enjoy better public health and have higher health indicators. Democracies are more invested in their human capital (Baum and Lake 2003) and are more concerned with public opinion than autocratic regimes. Consequently, democratic governments are likely to place a higher priority on health care. The *POLITY Score* variable reflects the level of democracy in a state.[10]

As in the analysis of HALE, levels of national income are expected to be related to higher levels of public health. States with greater wealth will have greater resources for health expenditures than poorer states. The populations of wealthier states will, therefore, enjoy higher life expectancies and have lower fertility and infant mortality rates. The *Per-Capita GDP* (gross domestic product) variable is the real GDP of a state. Economic openness will have a similar effect on the selected measures of public health as trade may act as a significant generator of revenue. Moreover, trade reflects ties with the larger international community, which could lead to external

Table 5.1. Summary Statistics

Variables	Mean	Standard Deviation	Minimum	Maximum
Dependent Variables				
Fertility Rate	3.94	2.03	1.09	10.13
Infant Mortality Rate	57.30	51.92	2.6	263
Male Life Expectancy	59.43	11.32	30	77.32
Female Life Expectancy	64.01	12.79	32.5	84.11
Independent Variables				
Year	1980.28	11.99	1960	1999
Lagged Major Conflict	0.06	0.25	0	1
Lagged Major Conflict Duration	0.46	2.82	0	40
Lagged Minor Conflict	0.08	0.27	0	1
Lagged Minor Conflict Duration	0.71	3.70	0	40
Lagged POLITY score	−0.44	7.55	−10	10
Lagged ln(Population)	15.32	1.91	10.61	20.95
Lagged ln(Per-Capita GDP)	7.47	1.53	4.34	10.81
Lagged ln(Trade Openness)	4.04	0.64	0.35	6.08

NOTE: Number of observations varies across models.

pressure for or assistance in maintaining adequate health care systems. The *Openness* variable reflects trade as a proportion of GDP.[11] I also expect population size to have a positive relationship with health levels. A smaller proportion of larger populations gets affected by natural disasters, diseases, and war. Consequently, the effect of many factors that reduce health achievement is less significant in states where a large percentage of the population may not be affected.[12] All the independent variables, except *Year*, are lagged to better account for the effect of time. *Per-Capita GDP*, *Openness*, and *Population* are logged. The summary statistics for these variables, as well as the dependent variables, are shown in Table 5.1.

In the following sections, I analyze the effect of conflict and the other covariates on fertility rates, infant mortality rates, male life expectancy, and female life expectancy.

FERTILITY RATES

The total fertility rate of a state represents the average number of children women in that population bear during their reproductive years. At a replacement fertility rate of 2.1, a population will remain stable if no immigration or emigration occurs. Above this rate, a population will increase, and below

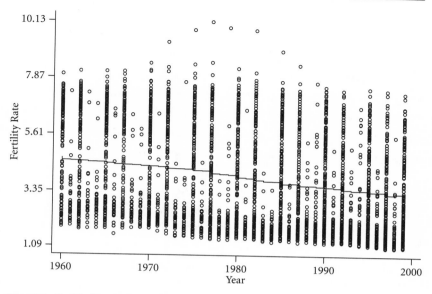

Figure 5.1. Fertility Rates, 1960–1999

this rate, there will be an eventual decrease in population. Figure 5.1 shows the global trend in fertility rates between 1960 and 1999.

In the past few decades, fertility rates in many parts of the world—particularly in developed countries—have been declining. The global decline in fertility rates began in the late 1950s and continued in subsequent decades in most parts of the world, except in sub-Saharan Africa and a number of Arab countries (Caldwell 2001). The factors contributing to lower fertility rates across the world include higher life spans due to improvements in health care, government policies aimed at population control, access to contraception, and a rise in economic opportunities for women. In his explanation of the demographic transition toward lower mortality and declining fertility rates, Cleland (2001) states:

> Nearly all classical representations of demographic transition depict the following chronological sequence: a fall in death rates, an ensuing period of rapid natural increase, a lagged decline of birth rates, and an eventual return to population equilibrium. ... Within this framework, the structural modernization of societies acts as the common cause of both mortality and fertility decline. (60)

Some of the socioeconomic factors leading to this transition are "changing costs and benefits of children, new economic roles for women, and the erosion of the family as a productive unit" (Cleland 2001, 60).

Provision of improved health care leads to longer life expectancies and, therefore, increases the number of people to be supported by the family as well as the society at large. This necessitates population control through limiting birthrates in order for societies to continue to meet their public health and economic goals. Families' accessibility to adequate contraception and preventive health care is imperative in implementing government policies as well as couples' choices regarding fertility rates (Tsui and Bogue 1978; Tsui 2001; Bacci 2001). Tsui (2001) assesses the impact of state policies on fertility rates and describes lower fertility rates as a "public good," particularly in poorer regions of the world. She outlines three types of organized efforts by states to control birthrates: extensive national boards for family planning, state supervision of maternal and child health, and private or nonprofit organization for family planning advice.

> Countries that have all three types of provider groups, as well as an active commercial sector, are perceived as having strong national effort. In other countries where contraceptive imports may be embargoed and local manufacturing is nil, where the public health program does not provide contraceptives, or where only a local family planning affiliate in the capital is operative, the national effort is considered weak. (187–188)

Involvement of states in violent conflict is likely to have a negative effect on the states'—as well as private organizations'—ability to engage in widespread provision of contraceptives to the population. Moreover, women are less likely to have the economic opportunities that might enable them to make reproductive choices. As a result, conflict may lead to increased fertility rates.

I evaluate the effect of war on fertility rates through a country-specific fixed effects model; the data on fertility rates were obtained from the World Bank's *World Development Indicators* (World Bank 2004). Table 5.2 shows the results for the model assessing the influence of war and relevant socioeconomic factors on fertility rates in all countries between 1960 and 1999.

Table 5.2. The Effect of Conflict on Fertility Rates, 1960–1999

Variables	All Regions	Africa	Asia	Europe/ North America	Latin America	Middle East
(Constant)	66.13	60.22	60.92	62.11	117.42	327.37
	(3.25)	(17.35)	(14.86)	(3031)	(8.86)	(19.34)
Year	−0.02	0.01	0.00	−0.02**	−0.04**	−0.18**
	(<0.01)	(0.01)	(0.01)	(<0.01)	(0.01)	(0.01)
Lagged Major Conflict	−0.13	0.03	−0.32	−0.27	−0.31	0.41
	(0.07)	(0.3)	(1.19)	(1.14)	(0.14)	(0.25)
Lagged Major Conflict Duration	0.02	0.01	0.04	0.13	0.04	0.03
	(0.01)	(0.02)	(0.07)	(0.14)	(0.02)	(0.06)
Lagged Minor Conflict	−0.27	−0.37	−0.15	−0.16	0.09	−0.40
	(0.06)	(0.23)	(0.11)	(0.10)	(0.14)	(0.15)
Lagged Minor Conflict Duration	0.02**	0.03	−0.01	0.01	−0.04	0.07**
	(<0.01)	(0.02)	(0.02)	(0.01)	(0.01)	(0.01)
Lagged POLITY score	−0.02**	−0.01**	−0.02**	−0.02**	0.01	−0.05**
	(<0.01)	(<0.01)	(<0.01)	(<0.01)	(<0.01)	(0.02)
Lagged ln(Population)	−1.75**	−1.77**	−3.27**	−1.41**	−2.53**	1.56
	(0.09)	(0.43)	(0.43)	(0.19)	(0.27)	(0.33)
Lagged ln(Per-Capita GDP)	−0.42**	−0.31**	−0.33*	−0.23**	−0.01	1.12
	(0.05)	(0.10)	(0.14)	(0.07)	(0.13)	(0.17)
Lagged ln(Trade Openness)	−0.18**	0.13	−0.21*	−0.29**	−0.06	−0.18
	(0.05)	(0.09)	(0.09)	(0.06)	(1.11)	(0.12)
F−test(FE)	76.81	18.34	55.33	82.22	35.10	63.18
ρ	0.97	0.97	0.99	0.98	0.98	0.97
N	2,417	523	292	1,012	379	211

NOTE: Cell entries are coefficient estimates; numbers in parentheses are robust standard errors. * = $p < .05$; ** = $p < .01$ (one-tailed).

I also present the results of this model for specific regions. During the period studied, fertility rates declined significantly in Europe and North America,[13] Latin America, and the Middle East. However, the presence of conflict does not have a significant impact on fertility rates in any specific region. The duration of minor conflict increases fertility rates in the model with all regions. And this effect is also significant in the Middle East, where minor conflicts have been protracted over decades. For instance, the total fertility rate of the Palestinian population between 1991 and 1995 was estimated at 7.73, which, Fargues (2000) argues, is a "corollary of the long-lasting state of belligerence between Arab Palestinians and Jews that began in the wake of the Balfour Declaration of 1917" (441). Rising sentiments of nationalism among the Palestinian population, a desire to give birth to more boys to carry on the fight, and expected loss of life due to the conflict, have resulted in high fertility rates.

As hypothesized, democracy is negatively related to fertility rates globally as well as in all the regions, except Latin America. Liberal democratic regimes are more invested in the quality of life of their populations and are, therefore, more likely to take measures to instigate and implement policies of population control. Since democracies are expected to enjoy higher levels of health achievement, they are likely to have higher life expectancies. As people live longer, it becomes important to limit fertility rates in order to avoid population increases to a level that cannot be supported adequately by society. Moreover, democratic states tend to have female representation in their governmental institutions, offering women a voice in reproductive decisions and possibly leading to widespread access to contraception.

States with larger populations are likely to have lower fertility rates. This result is in the hypothesized direction and holds for all countries and regions, with the exception of the Middle East. Large population size will induce states to implement rigorous family planning programs and focus on policies for population control. As populations grow, governments become cognizant of the possible effect on resources and undertake measures to limit birthrates. In 1951, India and China, due to their rapidly growing populations, were among the first countries to adopt a national population policy (Tsui 2001). Higher levels of national income are also associated with lower fertility rates, except in Latin America. Wealthier states are able to offer better health provisions to their populations, which include contraceptives and information on family planning. Consequently, people have the ability to make informed decisions about reproduction. Bacci (2001) asserts that "insufficient command over reproduction by women and men" (283) is one of the main reasons for fertility rates exceeding the desired family size of couples. Trade openness is also related to lower fertility rates in the world, as well as in Asia, Europe, and North America.

INFANT MORTALITY RATES

The second measure of public health to be assessed is infant mortality rates. Infant mortality rate is an important determinant of family health and is reported as deaths per 1,000 live births. As an indicator of improved health care in most of the world, infant mortality rates have been declining steadily in the past half-century. Figure 5.2 shows the global trend in infant mortality rates between 1960 and 1999.

According to World Health Organization (2000) estimates, worldwide infant mortality rates declined from 150 per 1,000 live births in 1950 to 68 in 1990. Adequate maternal, reproductive, and family health is necessary for low infant mortality rates. Widely accepted factors that influence infant mortality rates include health care and health technology, sanitation, nutrition, clean water, and economic resources (Rodgers 1979; Flegg 1982). Illiteracy and education of mothers is also considered an influence on mortality rates as women who can read are better informed about health choices for themselves and their infants (Caldwell 1979; Flegg 1982). Population scholars have also examined linkages between fertility and infant mortality rates and generally expect a direct relationship between the two. In societies with higher infant mortality, fertility rates are likely to be higher to compensate for actual or expected infant or child deaths. As infant mortality decreases, population control measures become more effective. Conversely, high fertility rates may cause higher infant mortality rates due to questionable maternal health and closely spaced births (Flegg 1982).

I examine the effect of war and the same covariates used in the previous models, but using infant mortality rates as a measure of population health.

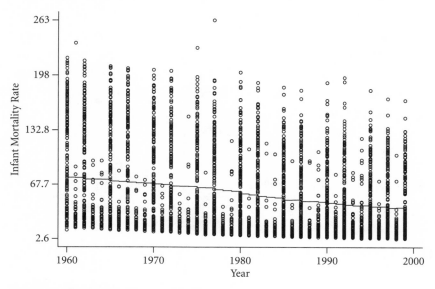

Figure 5.2. Infant Mortality Rates, 1960–1999

I expect involvement in war to have a positive effect on infant mortality rates, thus contributing to a deterioration in public health. The data on infant mortality rates come from the *World Development Indicators* (World Bank 2004). Table 5.3 shows the results for a fixed effects model for all countries between 1960 and 1999. The analysis reveals that infant mortality rates have decreased globally during this period, as well as in specific regions. The decline in infant mortality rates may be attributed to improved technology, provision of better health care, an increased number of births in hospitals, and higher levels of maternal health. Although the effect of time is consistent across the world, the effects of the other explanatory variables differ across regions.

Among the conflict variables, *Major Conflict Duration* and *Minor Conflict Duration* have a significantly positive relationship with infant mortality rates. This indicates that in the year following a major conflict, the number of infant deaths is likely to increase. A minor conflict, on the other hand, does not increase infant mortality unless it becomes protracted and lasts for a longer duration. However, these relationships are not statistically significant

Table 5.3. The Effect of Conflict on Infant Mortality Rates, 1960–1999

Variables	All Regions	Africa	Asia	Europe/ North America	Latin America	Middle East
(Constant)	1,570.33	2,856.78	2,059.51	437.07	2,973.97	5,164.88
	(63.90)	(383.35)	(248.95)	(47.46)	(171.09)	(398.94)
Year	−0.26**	−1.20**	−0.46**	−0.14**	−1.16**	−2.34**
	(0.06)	(0.27)	(0.18)	(0.03)	(0.12)	(0.26)
Lagged Major Conflict	4.19**	2.60	−1.49	−5.50	0.39	−2.98
	(1.38)	(5.60)	(3.02)	(3.78)	(2.78)	(4.62)
Lagged Major Conflict Duration	−1.30	−0.67	0.45	3.05	−0.34	−0.76
	(0.23)	(0.54)	(1.06)	(2.09)	(0.39)	(1.19)
Lagged Minor Conflict	−5.32	9.03	−3.44	−2.85	−5.61	−17.32
	(1.09)	(5.17)	(1.80)	(1.48)	(2.93)	(3.40)
Lagged Minor Conflict Duration	0.67**	−0.56	−0.22	0.15	−0.34	2.59**
	(0.11)	(0.44)	(0.42)	(0.16)	(0.30)	(0.16)
Lagged POLITY score	−0.40**	0.22	−0.49**	−0.63**	−0.08	−.30
	(0.05)	(0.12)	(0.12)	(0.04)	(0.10)	(0.34)
Lagged ln(Population)	−60.00**	−21.79*	−64.62**	1.73	−43.55**	−18.52**
	(1.73)	(9.42)	(7.33)	(2.68)	(5.14)	(6.75)
Lagged ln(Per Capita GDP)	−3.90**	−0.55	7.10	−16.14**	3.32	−22.20**
	(0.99)	(2.26)	(2.31)	(0.94)	(2.55)	(3.53)
Lagged ln(Trade Openness)	−3.22**	−6.43**	−2.76	−5.26**	8.51	0.27
	(.088)	(1.99)	(1.55)	(0.79)	(2.32)	(0.21)
F–test (FE)	102.63	48.73	150.42	89.27	56.84	37.44
ρ	0.99	0.94	0.99	0.97	0.98	0.94
N	2,478	528	310	1,014	391	235

NOTE: Cell entries are coefficient estimates; numbers in parentheses are robust standard errors. * = $p < .05$; ** = $p < .01$ (one-tailed).

in the region-specific models. It is particularly surprising that the duration of major conflict does not affect infant mortality rates. This counterintuitive finding may reflect the possibility that during protracted conflicts, populations adjust to societal conditions and appropriately guard against infant mortality. Consequently, as the conflict perpetuates, the increase in infant mortality caused by major conflict during the first year is addressed by societies through capacity building and resource allocation.

Levels of democracy are associated with lower infant mortality rates in the world, in Asia, and in Europe and North America. This supports the expectation that democracies provide superior health care to their populations and enjoy higher levels of public health than nondemocratic states. Democracy, however, does not have a significant effect on infant mortality rates in Africa, Latin America, and the Middle East. The effect of population size is in the hypothesized direction. Larger populations are associated with lower infant mortality rates. This result holds globally and for all the regions except Europe and North America, where population size has no effect on infant mortality. Higher levels of national income have a negative effect on infant mortality rates in the world, as well as in Europe, North America, and the Middle East. Surprisingly, GDP is not related to infant mortality in Africa, Asia, and Latin America. Rodgers (1979) and Flegg (1982) argue that income inequality is a major influence on infant mortality rates. The regions in which national income does not negatively affect infant mortality—Africa, Asia, and Latin America—also suffer from considerable inequalities in the distribution of income and wealth. Thus, it is possible that as GDP rises, only a certain proportion of the population benefits. Economic openness is inversely related to infant mortality rates in the world, in Africa, in Latin America, in Europe, and in North America.

LIFE EXPECTANCY

Life expectancy is the single most consulted measure of public health. Total life expectancy at birth is the average number of years that a person can expect to live at the current mortality rate of the population. Specifically, it is the average number of years that a group of people born in the same year are expected to live, if future mortality at each age remains constant. Life expectancy at birth indicates the level of health in a society and thus reflects the quality of life enjoyed by its members. However, total life expectancy only takes mortality into consideration and does not account for nonfatal health outcomes, including disease and disability or quality of life. HALE, on the other hand, is a measure of life years expected to be spent in full health and is thus a more appropriate measure of population health (see Chapter 4). But data on the HALE measure have only been calculated since 1999; total life expectancy estimates are available for a longer period.

I argue that war, through its direct and indirect effects, leads to a decline in life expectancy. This section applies the same models used to assess the effect of war on fertility and infant mortality rates to total life expectancy. Two separate models are estimated for male and female life expectancies; conflict may influence the well-being of men and women in a different manner. I use the *World Development Indicators* (World Bank 2004) for data on male and female life expectancies.

Male Life Expectancy

Male life expectancy at birth refers to the average number of years men are expected to live given the current mortality rates for men in a population. In the data used in this analysis, the lowest male life expectancy was 30 years, which was in Cambodia in 1977. The highest male life expectancy was 77.32, which was in Japan in 1999. As part of an overall global trend toward better population health, also manifested by declining fertility and infant mortality rates, male life expectancy has been increasing since 1960. This trend is shown in Figure 5.3.

The results for the fixed effects model evaluating the effects of war on male life expectancy are shown in Table 5.4. As in the previous models, other independent variables include *Year, Democracy, Population, Per-Capita GDP,* and *Trade Openness.* This analysis reveals that male life expectancy has increased over time between 1960 and 1999 in all regions of the world, as is shown by the significant coefficient on *Year.* This is consistent with the general trends toward better global health, including lower fertility and infant mortality rates. Improvements in medicine, increased access to health care, higher levels of knowledge about health issues, and better nutrition

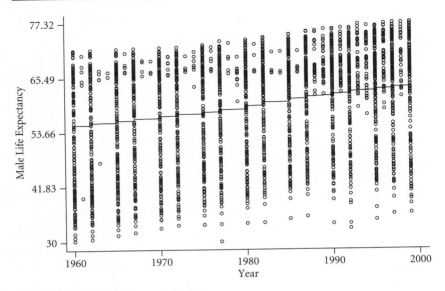

Figure 5.3. Male Life Expectancy, 1960–1999

have led to higher life expectancies in most of the world. It is important to note, however, that in spite of the rise in male life expectancy levels across the world, there are enormous global inequalities in levels of health and mortality. In 1999, the most recent year in this analysis, male life expectancy was 36 years in Sierra Leone and 77.32 years in Japan. Sierra Leone's low male life expectancy may be attributed to years of civil war, high HIV/AIDS rates, and persistent poverty. The per-capita GDP in Sierra Leone decreased from $219 in 1960 to $138 in 1999.

The occurrence of major conflict, as expected, leads to a decrease in male life expectancy in the model for all countries and regions. The direct casualties of war and deaths resulting from conflict-induced disease, famine, and displacement affect the conditions of mortality and longevity. The models for specific regions do not reveal this relationship, and a negative effect of minor conflict on male life expectancy is evident only for Africa. Although the duration of major conflict does not seem to be significantly related to the life expectancy of men, the duration of minor conflict does have a negative effect on male life expectancy in the global model and in the Middle

Table 5.4. The Effect of Conflict on Male Life Expectancy, 1960–1999

Variables	All Regions	Africa	Asia	Europe/North America	Latin America	Middle East
(Constant)	-303.75	-405.43	-459.72	-278.90	-384.32	-697.24
	(16.32)	(95.90)	(44.41)	(12.90)	(35.05)	(57.88)
Year	0.12**	0.23**	0.17**	0.13**	0.15**	0.32**
	(0.01)	(0.07)	(0.03)	(0.01)	(0.03)	(0.04)
Lagged Major Conflict	-0.91**	2.02	0.06	1.81	-0.77	0.05
	(0.33)	(1.39)	(0.54)	(1.01)	(0.57)	(0.70)
Lagged Major Conflict Duration	0.17	0.01	-0.27	-0.83	0.08	-021
	(0.05)	(0.14)	(0.20)	(0.52)	(0.08)	(0.18)
Lagged Minor Conflict	0.78	-3.31**	0.21	0.38	0.64	2.08
	(0.27)	(1.29)	(0.33)	(0.44)	(0.60)	(0.49)
Lagged Minor Conflict Duration	-0.07*	0.11	0.08	0.02	0.02	-0.36**
	(0.03)	(0.11)	(0.07)	(0.04)	(0.06)	(0.03)
Lagged POLITY score	-0.01	-0.13	0.03	-0.04	-0.01	0.04
	(0.01)	(0.03)	(0.02)	(0.01)	(0.02)	(0.04)
Lagged ln(Population)	7.51**	-0.01	10.20**	4.83**	10.36**	6.80**
	(0.43)	(2.36)	(1.27)	(0.78)	(1.09)	(0.97)
Lagged ln(Per-Capita GDP)	1.89**	-0.68	0.58	1.51**	-0.32	3.88**
	(0.23)	(0.56)	(0.42)	(0.25)	(0.52)	(0.50)
Lagged ln(Trade Openness)	0.27	1.28*	0.14	0.25	-1.26	-1.73
	(0.21)	(0.50)	(0.28)	(0.21)	(0.47)	(0.35)
F–test (FE)	93.17	26.76	134.52	128.71	71.94	65.63
ρ	0.98	0.82	0.99	0.99	0.99	0.99
N	1,945	518	248	637	342	200

NOTE: Cell entries are coefficient estimates; numbers in parentheses are robust standard errors. $* = p < .05$; $** = p < .01$ (one-tailed).

East. This finding is consistent with the likelihood of higher fertility and infant mortality rates in the Middle East due to prolonged minor conflict. The duration of minor conflict is associated with a deterioration of health outcomes in the Middle East to a greater degree than in other regions. In contrast to the other measures of population health, male life expectancy does not seem to be related to levels of democracy. Democracy does have a significantly positive effect on male life expectancy in a bivariate analysis of the relationship, but this effect disappears once the model controls for *Year*. Population, on the other hand, has a positive relationship with male life expectancy worldwide and in all the regions, except Africa, and this finding is in the hypothesized direction. Larger populations may enjoy increased public health resources, including a larger pool of human capital from which health care personnel can be recruited. Life expectancy for men is likely to benefit from higher levels of GDP per capita at the global level and in Europe, North America, and the Middle East. Trade openness has a positive effect on male life expectancy only in Africa.

Female Life Expectancy

The total female life expectancy at birth refers to the average number of years women in a population are expected to live if the current mortality conditions remain constant. It is "the number of years a newborn infant would live if prevailing patterns of age-specific mortality rates at the time of birth were to stay the same throughout the child's life" (United Nations Development Programme 2003, 354). Similar to male life expectancy, female life expectancy has also increased between 1960 and 1999, and this trend is displayed in Figure 5.4.

The rise in female life expectancy reflects improvements in nutrition, education, medicine, and health care in most of the world. During the past few decades, female life expectancy has been a little higher than male life expectancy. In the sample for this analysis, the mean female life expectancy is 1.47 years higher than the average male life expectancy. There is no consensus on the reasons for the difference between life expectancy for men and women, but possible reasons include gender differences in employment conditions and in habits regarding eating, drinking, and smoking. Men are

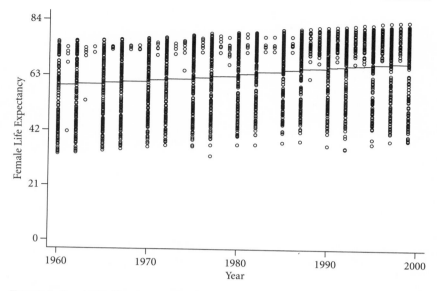

Figure 5.4. Female Life Expectancy, 1960–1999

more likely than women to work under hazardous conditions, such as in combat or in factories. In many societies, men are more likely to be exposed to violence and murder.

I assess the effect of war on female life expectancy with an analysis similar to the models used to examine the relationship between conflict and fertility rates, infant mortality rates, and male life expectancy. The data for female life expectancy were also obtained from the *World Development Indicators* (World Bank 2004) and the results for the analysis are reported in Table 5.5. Not surprisingly, the results for the analysis of female life expectancy are not tremendously different from the models evaluating male life expectancy. Most of the factors influencing life expectancy affect men and women in a similar manner. The negative effect of major conflict on male life expectancy, however, is not evident for female life expectancy. This may be the result of higher male exposure to the direct effects of war. Most militaries are composed entirely of men and combat, therefore, is likely to generate more male than female casualties. Minor conflict has a negative effect on female life expectancy in Africa and the duration of minor conflict

Table 5.5. The Effect of Conflict on Female Life Expectancy, 1960–1999

Variables	All Regions	Africa	Asia	Europe/ North America	Latin America	Middle East
(Constant)	−316.52	−470.26	−590.63	−257.60	−441.93	−818.06
	(18.51)	(112.07)	(48.63)	(10.92)	(30.32)	(61.31)
Year	0.12**	0.28**	0.25**	0.13**	0.17**	0.39**
	(0.01)	(0.08)	(0.03)	(0.01)	(0.02)	(0.04)
Lagged Major Conflict	−0.68	2.24	0.03	1.50	0.28	0.60
	(0.37)	(1.63)	(0.59)	(0.85)	(0.50)	(0.74)
Lagged Major Conflict Duration	0.20	0.02	−0.25	−0.78	0.08	−0.23
	(0.06)	(0.16)	(0.22)	(0.44)	(0.07)	(0.19)
Lagged Minor Conflict	0.93	−3.64*	0.30	0.53	1.41	2.06
	(0.31)	(1.50)	(0.37)	(0.37)	(0.52)	(0.51)
Lagged Minor Conflict Duration	−0.07*	0.12	0.09	−0.03	0.03	−0.37**
	(0.03)	(0.13)	(0.08)	(0.04)	(0.05)	(0.51)
Lagged POLITY score	<0.01	−0.15	0.02	0.02**	−0.02	0.08
	(0.01)	(0.04)	(0.02)	(0.01)	(0.02)	(0.05)
Lagged ln(Population)	7.45**	−2.71	8.91**	3.60**	11.76**	5.64**
	(0.49)	(2.75)	(1.39)	(0.66)	(0.96)	(1.03)
Lagged ln(Per Capita GDP)	2.43**	−0.48	0.55	1.95**	−0.31	3.93**
	(0.26)	(0.66)	(0.46)	(0.21)	(0.45)	(0.53)
Lagged ln(Trade Openness)	0.49*	1.53**	0.26	0.56**	−1.24	−1.76
	(0.24)	(0.58)	(0.31)	(0.17)	(0.40)	(0.37)
F-test (FE)	81.51	22.24	150.84	172.24	102.53	60.34
ρ	0.99	0.99	0.97	0.82	0.99	0.97
N	1,946	518	248	634	342	200

NOTE: Cell entries are coefficient estimates; numbers in parentheses are robust standard errors. $* = p < .05$; $** = p < .01$ (one-tailed).

decreases women's life expectancy in the Middle East. All the indicators of population health examined in this chapter are likely to suffer from protracted minor conflict in the Middle East. This is an interesting finding and it is consistent across all the models estimated in this chapter.

With respect to democracy, the models reveal a positive effect on female life expectancy only in Europe and North America. Similar to the models of male life expectancy, democracy does have a significantly positive effect on female life expectancy worldwide and in each region in bivariate analyses of the relationship. Controlling for *Year* eradicates the significance of this effect. The influence of population is also the same as for male life expectancy, that is, population size is positively related to female life expectancy globally and in all regions, expect Africa. National income is directly related to life expectancy of women globally, in North America, in Europe, and in the Middle East. The effect of trade openness is somewhat different here than in the analysis of male life expectancy. While male life expectancy increases due to trade only in Africa, female life expectancy is positively influenced by economic openness in Africa, Europe, and North America and to a lesser degree at the global level.

CONCLUSION

The analyses in this chapter provide mixed support for the proposed hypotheses regarding the effect of conflict on various measures of health. The impact of war on the chosen measures of population health—fertility rates, infant mortality rates, and male and female life expectancies—is not consistently significant in all the regions of the world. This indicates that our understanding of the relationship between war and health is far from comprehensive and continued efforts are required to extricate the complex mechanisms in this relationship. It is clear from these analyses, however, that the impact of conflict on health achievement varies across regions and indicators. Moreover, the intensity and duration of conflict affect regions and health indicators in a different manner.

One major issue in these analyses has been the quality of available data on health indicators. Unlike Health-Adjusted Life Expectancy (HALE) figures, the data on individual health indicators—such as infant mortality rates—do not reflect the overall level of health in a population. These dis-aggregated measures are employed due to their availability over a longer time period than HALE. However, in addition to not summarizing popula-tion health, the quality of these data are difficult to ascertain. First, there are considerable problems of missing data with most public health measures, particularly for developing countries. Second, there are cross-national com-parability issues due to different data collection and compilation methods used in various countries. Data from conflict-ridden societies are especially susceptible to quality-control issues, and quality issues specific to country-years with conflict might be impeding a clearer picture of the effect of war on health outputs.

In addition to the need for improvements in the quality of data, socio-economic factors not considered in these analyses might be driving some of the effects on health measures. The general effect of war on health in the models in this chapter is not as significantly negative as the hypotheses suggest. Hence, further research is needed to better understand how con-flict undermines the health of populations. For example, it is possible that inflows of international humanitarian aid during periods of conflict serve to mitigate some of the negative effects of violent conflict on public health. Significant international intervention and aid in states with previously low levels of health outcomes may result, for instance, in an increase in vaccina-tion programs and curative health provision. This is counterintuitive since the health care capabilities—particularly preventive care—of states are vis-ibly reduced in times of war; the intervening factor to explain maintenance of some aspects of health outputs may be international involvement.[14] Gov-ernmental and nongovernmental organizations—such as the Red Cross, the United Nations High Commissioner for Human Rights, and Doctors With-out Borders—establish and maintain a presence in war-ridden states, which mitigates the negative health impact of conflict. Humanitarian aid is often provided in conflicts that generate large refugee flows and the aid organiza-tions provide health care services to the refugee groups as well as the host populations. It is important to note that in bivariate analyses, all measures of violent conflict have the expected effect on each health indicator. The presence and duration of conflict significantly increase fertility and infant mortality rates and decrease life expectancy in both genders when models are estimated without controls.

Considerable evidence exists for the positive effect of democracy on public health. Populations of democratic states are likely to enjoy better health than those of nondemocratic states. Democratic regimes consider health care a higher priority than nondemocratic states due to a higher concern for public opinion; democracies also invest more in human capital (Baum and Lake 2003). Also, as expected, the analyses reveal a generally positive effect of national income on health. However, wealth is not related to higher life expectancy in Africa, Asia, and Latin America. These regions suffer from immense inequalities in wealth, which may be an explanation for the lack of a significant relationship between wealth and public health. Population experts and public health scholars consider income inequality within societies an important influence on certain health indicators, including fertility and mortality rates (Rodgers 1979; Flegg 1982; Wilkinson 1996; Kawachi et al. 1997). Shi (2002) finds that high levels of income inequality negatively affect health, even considering levels of democracy, which might explain the weak relationship between democracy and life expectancy in the analyses in this chapter. Enormous income inequalities might mean that most increases in GDP are limited to segments of society that already enjoy adequate health provisions. In order for health indicators for the entire society to improve due to rising national income, the income must be distributed throughout the population. This study does not test the effect of inequality on health, but it is important to note this influence on societal well-being.

On the one hand, the relationship between war and health is very simple. Wars kill people and destroy cities; clearly that is detrimental to the well-being of a society. On the other hand, the effect of conflict on health is rife with complex linkages since societal health is a function of myriad socioeconomic and political factors. A variety of domestic and international influences intervene in this relationship, and conflict may affect the health of societies through several different mechanisms. One important mechanism through which war undermines public health is the effect of armed conflict on key elements of a society's infrastructure. The next chapter examines linkages among violent conflict, infrastructure, and population health.

6

COLLATERAL DAMAGE: WAR, INFRASTRUCTURE, AND PUBLIC HEALTH

AS THE PREVIOUS CHAPTERS DEMONSTRATE, one of the most significant societal consequences of violent conflict—both at the intrastate and interstate levels—is its negative effect on the health achievement of states. Populations of states suffer short-term and long-term effects on their health and well-being as a result of every violent conflict in which their states become involved. The effect of conflict on population health, which reflects the human cost of war, is a significant component of the overall cost of conflict. Yet, save a few recent examinations (e.g., Ghobarah et al. 2003, 2004), the health consequences of war remain largely unexplored; much more attention has been paid to the political and economic consequences of war. Attention to the effects of war on public health is equally lacking in state-level policy making. To the extent that the human cost of war is taken into account while making conflict engagement decisions, the focus is limited to estimates of direct casualties of war. However, in addition to combat casualties, the health effects of war occur through a number of indirect mechanisms. Among the most important mechanisms through which conflict negatively impacts public health is the destruction of infrastructure, such as hospitals and transportation. In this chapter, I assess the impact of conflict-related damage to health-related and general infrastructure on key public health outputs.

The emphasis on the health consequences of conflict is consistent with the framework of human security, which calls for an evolution in the conceptualization of global and national security. The traditional approaches to the study of security focus chiefly on the state-level impact of conflict, including the effect on political institutions and specific regimes. The idea of security is generally limited to issues of sovereignty, and a state is considered secure if its national interests are safe from external aggression or unwelcome interference. Conversely, the notion of human security emphasizes the security of people within the borders of states (Annan 2000; Sen 2000; Thakur 1997; Bruderlein 2001). Although state security is a necessary condition for human security, it is far from a sufficient condition. The security of people is related to their quality of life and, therefore, the threats to their security include a range of social and economic issues. Components of human security include economic security, political security, access to food and health care, personal and community security, and environmental security (United Nations Development Programme 1994). Health is clearly an integral element of human security; health is in fact necessary for the enjoyment of any other aspects of human security. Threats to human health—such as disease, disability, high mortality rates, and low life expectancy—are major impediments to human security and tend to prevail during periods of violent conflict.

The effects of war on health occur through direct as well as indirect mechanisms through which the health achievement of a state declines with involvement in violent conflict; among the most important mechanisms through which conflict negatively influences public health is the effect on societal infrastrucure. In this chapter, I assess the impact of conflict on health outputs through its effects on key aspects of a society's infrastructure. Modern health care systems cannot be sustained without adequate infrastructure, which includes both the general infrastructure and health infrastrucure. The analysis in this chapter examines the linkages among conflict, indicators of infrastructure, and health achievement of states. I begin with a brief discussion of the significance of indirect means, such as infrastructure, through which war affects health. Then I describe the indicators I employ—for conflict, infrastructure, and health—in the empirical analysis. Finally, I present the analyses and discuss their findings.

CONFLICT, INFRASTRUCTURE, AND HEALTH

The most obvious and immediate way in which war undermines human security is through the deaths and disabilities that result from combat among the military and civilian populations. In addition to this direct impact of war, violent conflict may also affect public health through destruction of infrastructure, inability of states to provide basic services such as clean water and transportation, and a shortage in qualified health care personnel. Moreover, states may divert economic resources from social to defense spending and protracted conflicts may result in widespread poverty, crime, and gradual social decline; famines may also be associated with longer conflicts due to lower agricultural production. Conflict can also affect human security and population well-being through generations of refugee flows and large numbers of internally displaced persons. Although any kind of war can be linked to reduced health achievement, the negative effects of war on populations tend to be particularly severe in civil wars, in which the combat is focused on the territory of a single state; civil wars are also often marked by intense hatred between the opposing groups.

Interstate and intrastate conflict thus influence population health at several levels. Chapter 4 examined the direct effect of violent conflict on overall levels of population health in the short and the long term, and Chapter 5 assessed the impact of conflict on disaggregated measures of health. However, as mentioned above, the linkages between war and population well-being are complex; conflict undermines the health of populations through a number of indirect means. On the economic side, states may reduce the allocation of resources to public and health spending in favor of military expenditures to meet the heightened security needs of the state due to involvement in conflict (Russett 1982; Mintz and Huang 1991; Mintz 1989; Apostolakis 1992); these budgetary trade-offs may be accompanied by overall economic decline, particularly in protracted conflicts. I examine the economic effects of conflict in Chapter 7. Moreover, large groups of migrants during and after conflicts may be forced to live under conditions that are conducive to disease proliferation (Ghobarah et al. 2003); this dynamic will be discussed in Chapter 8.

In this chapter, I focus on damage to, and the deterioration of, a society's infrastructure as an indirect mechanism through which war leads to a decline in health levels. During violent conflict, damage to the general infrastructure may combine with a reduction in the capacity of the health care infrastructure at a time of increased health care needs. It is important to note that public health is affected not only by destruction of medical facilities but also by damage to elements of the larger infrastructure, such as transportation, the water supply, and power grids. For instance, during the Liberian crisis, the spread of cholera in the capital city of Monrovia could not be controlled due to the inability of Liberian and international agencies to conduct the necessary water chlorination processes (World Health Organization 2003).

War can damage both public health and the general infrastructure of a society; this damage to the infrastructure, at a time of increased health care needs, can be particularly devastating. Health care facilities and hospitals may be targeted during combat or may be rendered ineffective if their supply lines have been cut off due to the destruction of roads, bridges, and transportation networks. The Iraqi health care system was among the best in the region before the 1991 Gulf War but was nearly destroyed during the war. Health care in Iraq continued to decline rapidly—partly due to sanctions—during the subsequent decade. In 1993, Iraq's water supply was estimated at 50 percent of prewar levels (Hoskins 1997), and civilian deaths during and in the wake of the war reached 100,000 (Garfield and Neugut 1997).

The salient linkages among war, various elements of societal infrastructure, and the subsequent influence on population health and well-being drive the central questions of the analysis in this chapter. Figure 6.1 illustrates the conceptual framework for evaluating the direct and indirect effects of conflict on health; it depicts the key linkages among war, infrastructure, and public health. As Figure 6.1 shows, the challenge is to disentangle the direct effects of war on health from its indirect effects through degradation of a country's infrastructure. Note that the effect of war on health is twofold, both direct and through infrastructure. I also recognize other exogenous

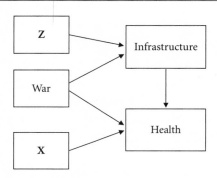

Figure 6.1. War, Infrastructure, and Health

factors directly influencing both health (denoted **X**) and infrastructure (denoted **Z**).[15]

In summary, I argue that despite the heightened ability of modern weapons to identify strategic targets, violent conflict damages key elements of a state's infrastructure. Some of these elements of infrastructure serve general purposes, such as roads and communications, while others are more specifically related to health care provision, including medical supplies and health care facilities. I assert that an impact on both categories of infrastructure has a detrimental effect on the health outcomes of a state, including broadly used measures of public health such as life expectancy and infant mortality. I assess the relationships among conflict, infrastructure, and health while accounting for other relevant influences on both infrastructure and public health—including the type of political institutions in a state and various economic factors. Next I discuss the indicators and data I include in the analysis, followed by empirical models that evaluate the hypothesized relationships.

DATA AND OPERATIONALIZATION

I analyze the effect of war on infrastructure and—indirectly through infrastructure—on public health for the period from 1960 to 2004. The models include all country-years during this period as the unit of analysis. The analysis contains four sets of variables: (1) the dependent variables indicating health achievement, (2) endogenous indicators of infrastructure that serve as the dependent variables in the first part of the analysis and covariates of health in the second, (3) the indicators of conflict as covariates of both infrastructure and health outputs, and (4) other relevant influences on infrastructure and/or health.

Health Achievement

As discussed in previous chapters, the most widely used and understood measure of public health is life expectancy, which is the number of years for which an average individual in a society is expected to live at birth. More nuanced summary measures of public health include Health-Adjusted Life Expectancy (HALE) and Disability-Adjusted Life Years (DALY), which account for years of life spent in less than full health (see Mathers et al. 2000). However, the data on these measures have only been collected by the World Health Organization (WHO) since 1998 and therefore limit our ability to identify long-term trends in health. The first indicator of public health I use in this analysis, therefore, is life expectancy, measured simply in life years. Life expectancy between 1960 and 2004 ranges from 23.68 years (Rwanda in 1992) to 81.80 years (Japan in 2004). I expect life expectancy to decrease with increased levels of violent conflict—both international and domestic—and with decreased levels of the infrastructure indicators. I also assess outputs of health by considering infant mortality rates. Infant mortality is measured by infant deaths per 1,000 live births; this variable is logged. During the period studied, the highest level of infant mortality was in Mali in 1960 (285 per 1,000) and the lowest was in Singapore in 2001 at 2.2 per 1,000. In 2004, the average infant mortality rate in sub-Saharan Africa was 100, with Sierra Leone's infant mortality rate being the highest in the region (and the world) at 165 per 1,000 live births. I expect infant mortality rates to increase at higher values of conflict engagement and lower values of infrastructure.

The third measure of public health in the analysis is fertility rates, which indicate the average number of children to whom women give birth in a population. Lower fertility rates reflect access to contraception, education on reproductive issues, and attention to women's health. Consequently, lower fertility rates are associated with higher levels of general and reproductive health. In this analysis, the lowest fertility rate is 0.84 (China in 2002) and the highest is 8.5 (Rwanda in 1982). As with other indicators of public health, fertility rates are likely to worsen (that is, increase) due to involvement in conflict and reduced infrastructural capacity. The data for all three health-related dependent variables were obtained from the World Bank's *World Development Indicators* (2006).

Infrastructure

The choice of indicators for various elements of infrastructure was severely limited due to data availability issues. Within availability constraints, I employ two measures of health-related infrastructure and two measures of general infrastructure that serve the health sector as well as the society at large. The data for all four variables were acquired from *World Development Indicators* (World Bank 2006).

Health Infrastructure   I use measures of immunization for DPT (diphtheria, pertussis, and tetanus) and measles in a given population as indicators of health infrastructure; these variables measure the percentage of children in a population who have received these vaccinations. Provision of immunizations is an appropriate indicator of health infrastructure as it reflects a functioning health care system. It is important to note that immunizations are a key element of preventive—and not curative—health, thus reflecting the level of national commitment to public health. Widespread provision of immunizations also requires health care facilities and clinics, relevant medical supplies, transportation, accessibility, and trained personnel. I expect both DPT and measles immunizations to be negatively related to incidence of violent conflict, and I expect reductions in immunizations to lead to a reduction in public health as measured by the three indicators described above.

General Infrastructure   To assess general infrastructure, I use one measure related to transportation and the other to communication. The former is a measure of paved roads in a state and the latter is the number of telephones (both mobile and land lines) per 1,000 people in a population. Due to the large discrepancy between telephone subscriptions in the developed countries and those in lesser developed regions, this variable is logged. Transportation and communications are useful to the entire society and are necessary for adequate health provision. I expect both of these indicators of general infrastructure to be negatively affected by a state's involvement in conflict and reductions in the levels of these variables to decrease health achievement.

Conflict

I assess the effect of both interstate and civil conflict on the selected indicators of infrastructure as well as on health outcomes. To measure conflict, I use the Armed Conflict Dataset compiled by the Peace Research Institute of Oslo (PRIO; Gleditsch et al. 2002). For both types of conflict, each country year has a value ranging from zero to three. Zero represents absence of any conflict, one reflects a minor conflict, two indicates intermediate conflict, and three denotes intense conflict. The PRIO definitions for minor, intermediate, and major conflict are retained (see Strand et al. 2005). As discussed above, I expect conflict to negatively affect both infrastructure and health. The effect of conflict on health is expected to occur both directly as well as through the deterioration of infrastructure. Since the effect of conflict on either infrastructure or health is not expected to be contemporaneous, both conflict variables are lagged one year. During the period under consideration, there were 840 internal conflicts of varying intensities and 280 interstate conflicts. Although I expect both types of conflict to affect infrastructure and health negatively, I expect this effect to be greater for civil wars due to the devastation often associated with domestic conflicts. International conflicts that are limited to border areas may have lower societal effects than civil wars that occur within the territory of a state.

Other Covariates

A number of expected determinants of infrastructure and health are included in the analysis. The first is a state's regime type. It is generally believed that democracies are more concerned about the welfare of their populations, have higher levels of health expenditures, and invest relatively more in human capital than nondemocratic regimes (see Baum and Lake 2003). Consistent with these arguments, I expect levels of democracy to be

Table 6.1. Summary Statistics

Variables	Observations	Mean	Standard Deviation	Minimum	Maximum
Health Achievement					
Life Expectancy	4,545	64.32	11.48	23.68	81.80
ln(Infant Mortality)	2,789	3.28	1.12	0.79	5.65
Fertility Rates	4,880	3.65	1.97	0.84	8.5
Infrastructure					
DPT Immunization	4,438	73.29	25.05	0	99
Measles Immunization	4,331	71.85	24.23	0	99
ln(Telephones)	5,811	3.86	1.95	−2.15	7.60
Paved Roads	1,977	49.51	33.20	0.8	100.1
Conflict					
Lagged Internal Conflict	6,155	0.28	0.76	0	3
Lagged International Conflict	6,155	0.11	0.52	0	3
Other Covariates					
POLITY score	5,683	−0.32	7.66	−10	10
ln(GDP)	6,779	8.30	1.14	5.14	11.34
GDP Growth	6,658	2.00	7.72	−63.32	151.06
ln(Openness)	6,789	4.07	0.75	0.70	6.90
Government Spending	6,779	22.30	11.26	1.53	93.72
Year (1960 = 0)	11,003	22.03	13.50	−1	45

positively related to health outcomes. I also expect democratic states to have higher levels of infrastructure; democratic leaders have greater incentives to invest in public works as their election/reelection rests on the approval of the larger electorate rather than on a small elite or selectorate (Bueno de Mesquita et al. 2003). As a result, indicators of infrastructure, such as immunizations and roads, are likely to be higher for democratic states. The *POLITY score* variable reflects the regime type of a state as measured by its POLITY IV score (Marshall and Jaggers 2004).

Some relevant economic variables are also included in the analysis. These are per-capita gross domestic product (GDP) in constant U.S. dollars, growth in national income, economic openness (imports and exports as a proportion of GDP), and government spending as a percentage of GDP. I expect national income, growth in income, and openness to be positively related to both infrastructure and health. Government spending is expected to directly affect infrastructure (since most elements of infrastructure depend on state resources) and, through infrastructure, influence health outputs. The *Per-Capita GDP* and *Openness* variables are logged. Last, I include a variable for *Year* to account for the effect of time; the years are counted from 1960 to 2004. Summary statistics are presented in Table 6.1.

ANALYSIS AND RESULTS

In order to assess the direct and indirect effects of conflict on infrastructure and health, I employ a two-stage least squares model. The first stage of the analysis evaluates the effect of the covariates on the four indicators of infrastructure; these results are presented in Table 6.2. The analysis reveals that all indicators of infrastructure—health-related and general—have experienced higher levels over time, as indicated by the *Year* variable; this positive effect of time over the four decades studied is intuitive. Democracy—as measured by the *POLITY score*—has a positive effect on one indicator of health-related infrastrucure (DPT immunization) and one indicator of general infrastructure (telephones).

As expected, higher levels of national income are also associated with higher levels of infrastructure, as measured by all four variables. It is hardly surprising that wealthier states enjoy better infrastructure. However, economic growth does not significantly influence any indicator of infrastructure. This reflects that growing economies are not necessarily likely to immediately start investing in health and general infrastructure. By contrast, states with generally higher income levels are in a better position to allocate resources to infrastructure. Economic openness is associated with higher levels of DPT immunization and paved roads but not the other two variables. And government spending has a positive effect on both DPT and measles immunizations as well as paved roads. For instance, a one-percentage-point increase in government spending leads to a 0.23 percent increase in DPT immunization and a 0.28 percent increase in measles immunization at the national level. The absence of a significant effect of government spending on telephone subscriptions is completely understandable since most telephones are acquired privately absent of state funds.

With respect to the effect of violent conflict, both DPT and measles immunization levels experience a decline if a state is involved in domestic

Table 6.2. Health and General Infrastructure

| | Health-Related | | General | |
Variables	DPT Immunization	Measles Immunization	Telephones	Paved Roads
Constant	−84.48	−76.96	−10.61	−169.89
	(5.65)	(5.85)	(0.19)	(14.02)
Lagged Internal Conflict	−2.30**	−2.16**	−0.05*	0.44
	(0.65)	(0.67)	(0.02)	(0.31)
Lagged International Conflict	0.29	0.02	−0.01	2.02
	(1.0)	(1.0)	(0.03)	(1.65)
Government Spending	0.23**	0.28**	0.02	0.56**
	(0.05)	(0.06)	(0.002)	(0.11)
POLITY score	0.17*	−0.01	0.04*	−0.09
	(0.08)	(0.08)	(0.003)	(−0.56)
ln(GDP)	11.54**	9.25**	1.49*	18.53**
	(0.52)	(0.54)	(0.02)	(1.03)
GDP Growth	0.08	0.005	−0.004	−0.09
	(0.07)	(0.07)	(0.002)	(0.13)
ln(Openness)	2.43**	0.63	−0.04	6.47**
	(0.8)	(0.82)	(0.03)	(1.66)
Year (1960 = 0)	1.44**	1.95**	0.05**	0.68*
	(0.08)	(0.10)	(0.002)	(0.32)
R^2	0.50	0.45	0.90	0.43
N	1,421	1,386	1,684	729

NOTE: Cell entries are two-stage least squares coefficient estimates; robust standard errors clustered by country are in parentheses. * = $p < .05$; ** = $p < .01$ (one-tailed).

conflict. A one-unit change in internal conflict results in a 2.3 percent reduction in DPT immunization. Given that the conflict variables range from zero for no conflict to three for intense conflict or war, this suggests that a civil war with more than 1,000 battle deaths in a year would reduce DPT immunization by nearly 7 percent. A similar effect exists for measles immunization. The number of telephones in a society also decreases due to civil conflict in the previous year, although the effect of domestic conflict on paved roads is not significant. Somewhat surprisingly, international conflict does not have a significant effect on the infrastructure indicators. This may suggest that international conflicts tend to occur in a more limited fashion—such as being restricted to state borders—than civil conflicts, thus explaining why the coefficient is not significant.

The second stage of the analysis disentangles the direct and indirect effects of war on the health indicators, shown in Tables 6.3, 6.4, and 6.5. These estimates indicate how war influences the various indicators of

Table 6.3. Life Expectancy

Variables	DPT Immunization	Measles Immunization	Telephones	Paved Roads
Constant	25.27	17.10	46.07	18.60
	(12.21)	(9.03)	(18.64)	(11.70)
Lagged Internal Conflict	0.443	0.224	−0.04	−0.33
	(0.53)	(0.49)	(0.43)	(0.56)
Lagged International Conflict	0.273	0.36	0.58	−0.005
	(0.28)	(0.31)	(0.38)	(0.31)
Infrastructure	0.32*	0.253*	4.75**	0.131*
	(0.16)	(0.13)	(1.84)	(0.075)
POLITY score	0.15*	0.21**	−0.005	0.21**
	(0.067)	(0.06)	(0.09)	(0.08)
ln(GDP)	3.86*	5.21**	0.73	5.01**
	(1.675)	(1.09)	(2.66)	(1.30)
GDP Growth	−0.04	−0.02	0.02	−0.014
	(0.04)	(0.04)	(0.03)	(0.03)
ln(Openness)	−1.34	−0.72	−0.53	−1.50
	(0.86)	(0.68)	(0.43)	(1.01)
Year (1960 = 0)	−0.37	−0.41	−0.14	0.10
	(0.24)	(0.25)	(0.10)	(0.08)
R	0.69	0.72	0.83	0.74
N	1,421	1,386	1,684	729

NOTE: Cell entries are two-stage least squares coefficient estimates; robust standard errors clustered by country are in parentheses. * $= p < .05$; ** $= p < .01$ (one-tailed).

public health as well as how infrastructure affects the health indicators; the effect of infrastructure on health incorporates the direct effect of conflict on infrastructure. The results for the models estimating the effects on life expectancy, infant mortality rates, and fertility rates are presented separately in Tables 6.3, 6.4, and 6.5, respectively.

Examining first the control variables, the analysis reveals that the *POLITY score* variable (democracy) has a positive effect on life expectancy in three of the four models that assess that measure of public health. Similarly, democracy positively affects—which is to say decreases—infant mortality rates in two of the models; fertility rates decrease (which indicates higher levels of health) with higher levels of democracy in three models as well. These results are consistent with previous arguments suggesting that population well-being levels are higher in democratic regimes; these results support the expectations in this study for the effect of democratic governance on health levels.

Table 6.4. Infant Mortality

Variables	DPT Immunization	Measles Immunization	Telephones	Paved Roads
Constant	8.14	8.77	3.91	7.40
	(1.38)	(1.03)	(2.89)	(3.06)
Lagged Internal Conflict	0.02	0.04	0.04	0.19*
	(0.06)	(0.06)	(0.04)	(0.09)
Lagged International Conflict	0.033	−0.006	0.01	0.11
	(0.03)	(0.03)	(0.04)	(0.08)
Infrastructure	−0.035*	−0.03*	−0.67*	−0.03
	(0.02)	(0.01)	(0.29)	(0.02)
POLITY score	−0.02**	−0.03**	0.01	−0.009
	(0.008)	(0.007)	(0.02)	(0.01)
ln(GDP)	−0.403*	−0.54**	0.18	−0.39
	(0.19)	(0.13)	(0.40)	(0.35)
GDP Growth	−0.004	−0.005	−0.009*	−0.01
	(0.004)	(0.004)	(0.004)	(0.007)
ln(Openness)	0.11	0.05	0.04	0.25
	(0.11)	(0.09)	(0.07)	(0.21)
Year (1960 = 0)	0.02	0.03	0.01	−0.02
	(0.02)	(0.02)	(0.01)	(0.01)
R^2	0.68	0.71	0.84	0.71
N	996	965	1,234	507

NOTE: Cell entries are two-stage least squares coefficient estimates; robust standard errors clustered by country are in parentheses. * = $p < .05$; ** = $p < .01$ (one-tailed).

As expected, the models also reflect a generally positive effect of national income—as measured by per-capita GDP—on the health variables. With a rise in national wealth, life expectancy increases in three of the four models, infant mortality decreases in two models, and fertility rates decrease in one model. The somewhat weak effect of GDP on fertility rates may be influenced by high birthrates in some very wealthy states—such as a number of the OPEC countries—as a result of either cultural factors or governmental incentives for population growth. Growth in GDP does not have a significant effect on health outcomes in most of the models. Economic growth does not increase life expectancy in any of the models, and it significantly decreases infant mortality and fertility rates only in one of the four models. Similarly, economic openness does not have a highly significant effect on any of the three measures of population health.

The model also indicates that the direct effects of conflict on health are not tremendously strong. Neither interstate nor intrastate conflict has

Table 6.5. Fertility Rates

Variables	DPT Immunization	Measles Immunization	Telephones	Paved Roads
Constant	8.87	10.31	4.27	8.43
	(2.84)	(2.07)	(5.26)	(2.84)
Lagged Internal Conflict	−0.03	0.01	0.06	0.08
	(0.11)	(0.11)	(0.09)	(0.15)
Lagged International Conflict	0.173*	0.15*	0.02	0.21*
	(0.08)	(0.08)	(0.13)	(0.10)
Infrastructure	−0.064*	−0.05*	−0.93*	−0.04**
	(0.04)	(0.03)	(0.52)	(0.02)
POLITY score	−0.054**	−0.06**	−0.03	−0.07**
	(0.016)	(0.015)	(0.03)	(0.015)
ln(GDP)	−0.357	−0.61**	0.24	−0.24
	(0.397)	(0.26)	(0.75)	(0.31)
GDP Growth	−0.005	−0.009	−0.02*	0.002
	(0.007)	(0.008)	(0.007)	(0.004)
ln(Openness)	0.33*	0.10	0.19	0.37
	(0.18)	(0.14)	(0.10)	(0.22)
Year (1960 = 0)	0.04	0.05	0.008	−0.06**
	(0.05)	(0.06)	(0.03)	(0.02)
R^2	0.62	0.63	0.79	0.61
N	1,508	1,469	1,805	753

NOTE: Cell entries are two-stage least squares coefficient estimates; robust standard errors clustered by country are in parentheses. * = $p < .05$; ** = $p < .01$ (one-tailed).

a significant direct effect on life expectancy. Internal conflict is associated with higher infant mortality rates in one model, while international conflict is associated with higher fertility rates in three models. This lack of strong direct effects suggests that the influence of war on health outcomes is occurring mainly through the instrumented infrastructure variables, all of which have significantly positive effects on all the measures of public health (with the exception of the effect of paved roads on infant mortality). Increases in all four indicators of infrastructure—DPT and measles immunizations, telephones, and paved roads—lead to substantial increases in life expectancy. For instance, a one-percentage-point increase in DPT immunization increases life expectancy by about four months, and a one-percentage-point increase in measles vaccination results in a three-month increase in life expectancy. Infant mortality rates decrease with higher levels of all infrastructure indicators, and fertility rates decline as three of the four infrastructure indicators increase in value. These findings support the assertion that infrastructure is an important mechanism through which violent conflict undermines the health and well-being of a society and, as expected, provide strong evidence for the linkages among war, societal infrastructure, and public health.

CONCLUSION

The analyses in this chapter evaluate one of many mechanisms through which war has the potential to undermine the health and well-being of populations. By examining the effect of conflict on health through infrastructural damage, this chapter illuminates the costs of war in terms of human security. However, estimating the complete human cost of war must involve assessment of both the direct impact of war and the many indirect mechanisms through which populations are affected during and after conflict.

Moreover, the impact of war on societal well-being—particularly through mechanisms such as infrastructure—is mediated to a great degree by states' ability to recover from conflict and the pace of post-conflict reconstruction. For instance, Western European states experienced some of their highest levels of health achievement after the end of World War II, which could be attributed to rapid reconstruction and an infusion of economic resources both through the Marshall Plan and internal economic growth. Conversely, conflict-ridden societies in sub-Saharan Africa, such as Rwanda and Sierra Leone, are much less able to recover from their wars. In terms of research on the human security costs of war, this suggests a need for attention to the long-term effects of conflict, particularly in lower-income and lesser-developed states. Of particular concern in this regard are the states of sub-Saharan Africa that have for decades been experiencing harrowing levels of conflict, poverty, and disease. In the next chapter, I assess the economic impact of violent conflict, particularly the budgetary trade-offs that result in diversion of resources from health spending to military expenditures.

7

THE ALLOCATION OF RESOURCES
BETWEEN DEFENSE AND HEALTH

IN CHAPTER 6, I examined the linkages among war, key elements of infrastructure, and specific indicators of public health. In this chapter, I evaluate another important mechanism through which conflict affects health. One way in which violent conflict leads to a deterioration in the public health provision of a state is through diversion of resources from social and health spending to military expenditures. Faced with pressing security concerns, states often prioritize defense spending over public health spending. These budgetary trade-offs result in obvious repercussions for public health, particularly as the health care needs of societies increase during times of violent conflict. This chapter tests the hypothesis that states lower their social spending and increase military spending due to involvement in armed conflict. States have access to a finite pool of resources that they must allocate among competing uses. The presence of militarized conflict compels states to reevaluate their resource allocation decisions in favor of military spending, and the increase in defense expenditures occurs at the expense of social spending, including resources used for public health. Consequently, the higher focus on national security may be related to lower levels of other important aspects of human security. I begin with a discussion of some theoretical and empirical work that assesses the relationship between levels of defense spending and various aspects of the economy. Next, I discuss the effect of conflict on these budgetary decisions, followed by an empirical analysis of the way in which conflict results in diversion of resources from social services and health to defense spending.

GUNS VERSUS BUTTER: THE EVIDENCE

The past three decades have seen a persistent scholarly interest in the economic cost of war and the determinants of defense spending. As states struggle with resource allocation decisions in an environment of limited availability of resources, they often have to make difficult choices among competing demands for expenditures. In a 1969 study, Russett raised the obvious yet potent question of who incurs the cost of defense in an economy, concluding that "guns do come at the expense of butter" (417) as increases in defense expenditures lead to decreases in personal consumption. His analysis also revealed that "America's most expensive wars have severely hampered the nation in its attempt to build a healthier and better-educated citizenry" (421). Since then, there have been a number of studies about defense spending and its impact on various sectors of the economy.

The investigations into the defense-welfare trade-offs have yielded mixed conclusions. Russett (1982) finds no evidence that either health or education spending was negatively related to defense expenditures in the United States between 1941 and 1979. However, Domke et al. (1983) find some evidence for guns-versus-butter trade-offs in an evaluation of long-term trends in advanced industrial democracies. Particularly during the Reagan years, the United States experienced extremely high levels of spending on defense and constraints on civilian spending (Mintz 1989). Assessing the effect of high defense expenditures on system leaders, Rasler and Thompson (1988) examine the position of Great Britain in the nineteenth century and the United States in the twentieth century. They evaluate the possibility that higher military expenditures, generally perceived as a source of global power and influence, could actually contribute to the decline of the power of world leaders. In addition to military might, economic growth and sustained prosperity are required for the status of world leadership. And if military expenditures occur at the expense of capital investment, they can lead to a decline in a systemic leader's power. Why then are capitalist economies willing to incur the high costs of defense spending? Due to their vulnerability to internal and external threats, capitalist political and economic systems must be protected by heightened defense budgets (Smith 1977). Similarly, a hegemonic world leader must defend the status quo of the entire system. Both Smith (1977) and Gilpin (1981) argue that the very military expenditures that hegemonic powers perceive as necessary for maintaining systemic status quo lead to a decline in their power.

Budgetary trade-offs between defense and civil uses are not limited to systemic leaders and are particularly important in small states with high levels of perceived security threats. As of 1984, Taiwan, South Korea, Brazil, Pakistan, Egypt, and Israel were allocating between 25 percent to 50 percent of their government expenditures to defense. Regional conflicts in the Third World have led to arms races, with consequent increases in defense spending (Mintz and Ward 1989). Fifty percent of all industrial investment in Israel occurs in the defense sector, 25 percent of the industrial labor force works in the defense sector, and some of the largest companies in Israel belong to this sector. Mintz and Ward (1989) argue that high levels of defense spending in Israel and other countries are a result of political and economic manipulation by sectors benefiting from the defense industry. Davis and Chan (1990), however, do not find either a positive or a negative impact of the defense expenditures of Taiwan on the island's social welfare indicators, presenting Taiwan as a deviant case for the study of defense-welfare spending. They attribute the lack of defense-welfare trade-off to Taiwan's strong human and physical capital, extensive U.S. aid, and a strategy of export-led growth. Ward et al. (1995) examine budgetary trade-offs in Japan and the United States from 1889 to 1991 and find that the existence and patterns of defense-growth trade-offs vary significantly in the two states and across time.

In Latin America, on the other hand, there is clear evidence for a guns-versus-butter trade-off. In his study of budgetary trade-offs in Latin America, Apostolakis (1992) argues that defense expenditures inevitably affect the allocation of resources to health, education, social security, and public works. His analysis reveals that military expenditures have been crowding out social spending through direct diversion of resources as well as an indirect effect through investment in Latin America in the short and the long term. In the case of Africa, it has been argued that governments allocate more resources to defense during times of austerity than during periods when the resources are increasing (Gyimah-Brempong 1992). This implies that defense spending increases at times when the society is most vulnerable due to lower levels of overall resources.

Mintz and Huang (1990) explore the social impact of higher levels of defense spending by evaluating the effect of military expenditures on investment and growth. They argue that increased levels of military spending have a negative effect on investment, and as defense spending goes down, investment levels rise. Since investment has an established positive effect on economic growth, higher levels of military spending are also linked to lower levels of growth. Testing their hypotheses about the effect of defense expenditures on investment and growth, Mintz and Huang (1990) find evidence of a direct as well as indirect effect of defense spending on economic growth through investment. They assert that this indirect trade-off between defense spending and economic growth begins to take effect in about a five-year period. Mintz and Huang (1991) also demonstrate a significant long-term indirect guns-verses-butter trade-off in the United States. Specifically, they show that the effect of military spending on growth through investment has a negative impact on education expenditures.

This is far from a comprehensive review of the studies on the guns-versus-butter debate, but this brief overview suggests the significance of budgetary trade-offs in resource allocation and their effect on societies. It also reflects the need for continued exploration of the ways in which states bear the cost of defense. Governments have a limited pool of resources to allocate among competing social and military needs, and the pressure for enhanced national security can lead to diversion of resources from civilian uses as well as affect society through repercussions for investment and growth.

The questions of interest in this chapter are whether and how the defense-welfare trade-off affects allocation of resources to public health and how this trade-off is influenced by violent conflict. The literature on budgetary trade-offs focuses primarily on studying the effects of defense spending on welfare but does not evaluate the direct effect of states' involvement in violent conflict on resource allocation decisions. Some studies mention increases in defense spending during times of war (e.g., Russett 1969), but the presence of conflict is not included as an independent variable in the models. In this chapter, I evaluate the effect of internal and international conflict on states' decisions to allocate economic resources to defense and social uses, particularly health. In the next section, I briefly discuss the economic cost of war and its relationship to public health.

CONFLICT, HEALTH, AND PUBLIC EXPENDITURES

Throughout history, wars have extracted heavy payments from societies, both in terms of economic resources and human suffering. Societies all over the world have had to divert resources from other uses, including health provisions, toward war efforts. During times of violent conflict, the monetary cost of defense can go up drastically, and states must meet this need by reallocating resources in favor of military expenditures. Wars need to be paid for, and the populations of states involved in conflict pay for war in terms of human capital as well as economic resources. Both developing and developed countries have important decisions to make about defense spending, particularly during times of conflict. Between 1960 and 1990, military expenditures increased about fourfold in constant U.S. dollars in developing countries. During the 1990s, per-capita military expenditures doubled in developing countries to facilitate larger armed forces, but there has been a decline in these expenditures in recent years. Although developed countries spend more on military expenditures in absolute terms, developing states cultivate higher defense spending burdens as a proportion of their gross domestic product (GDP), as well as in terms of human productivity (Levy and Sidel 2002).

An important aspect of defense spending is the international arms trade. The prevalent trend in arms trade is that industrialized states manufacture weapons and sell them to developing states. Due to the notion that building up an arms arsenal is a prerequisite for development, these developing states are compelled to purchase arms to maintain their regional power status.

Consequently, resources may be diverted from other, civilian uses, including public services. China, France, Russia, the United Kingdom, Germany, and the United States are the six largest arms exporters, supplying more than 90 percent of all international arms transfers. Annual arms imports tripled between 1960 and 1980, rising from US$14 billion in the early 1960s to US$35 billion in 1994 (Levy and Sidel 2002). In 1993, the United States was responsible for 47 percent of arms sales (in U.S. dollars), the United Kingdom made 20 percent of the sales, Russia had 12 percent, Germany 5 percent, France 4 percent, and China 4 percent. Fifty-eight percent of the imports went into developing countries and 42 percent into developed or industrialized states. However, only 7 percent of the exports were from developing countries; 93 percent came from industrialized states (Levy and Sidel 2002).

The extensive arms imports of developing countries have to be paid for somehow, and given the finite nature of economic resources, other aspects of the economy are likely to be affected. Since developing states are in greater need of improvements in social, health, and education services, the impact of purchasing arms is more detrimental for their societies than for the populations of developed states that have established social welfare and health care systems. It is interesting to note that a significant proportion of arms exports are made to nondemocratic states, which are more likely to divert resources from welfare to warfare since they are less constrained by public opinion than democracies. The economic costs of war and arms acquisition result in significant decline in health and human services, as well as damage to economic development. Particularly in developing states, higher levels of resources spent on military expenditures affect services such as education, public health, housing, and nutrition. Moreover, there are more general effects on development as the civilian sectors of the economy suffer at the expense of the defense sector.

Developing countries are more vulnerable to the deleterious effects of resource reallocation to defense expenditures. However, these effects also influence the societies of developed and industrialized states. Given that even developed states have finite resources, preparation for—and involvement in—conflict results in diversion of resources from civilian uses that would improve the quality of life of populations toward buildups of weapons arsenals. Such budgetary trade-offs were clearly demonstrated during the Reagan years (Mintz 1989). The Cold War witnessed significant reallocation of resources from welfare to war preparation in the United States. During that time, the Soviet Union spent an even higher percentage of its gross national product (GNP) on arms in order to match the dollar amounts spent by the United States. Between 1960 and 1981, the Soviet Union spent about 12 percent of its GDP on arms (Levy and Sidel 2002). This spending had a serious impact on social services and health expenditures.

Military spending by developed states also affects welfare and development in lesser-developed countries. Levy and Sidel (2002) note that:

> The amount that industrialized countries spend for military purposes indicates that they spend proportionately less on development assistance to developing countries. In 1989 the Scandinavian countries allocated around 1.0 percent of their GNP for official development assistance, as compared to 0.2 percent by the United States. ... Scandinavian countries and Japan allocated for official development assistance monies that ranged from 45 to 70 percent of their military expenditures, as compared to 3 percent for the United States. (217)

Hence, the negative effects of increased military expenditures may have global dimensions. Public health in developing countries is affected due to budgetary trade-offs their own governments make in favor of defense; these states also receive less in development aid from industrialized states due to their own higher military expenditures. As a result, the resources available for health care and preventive health decrease, the capacity of states to provide adequate public health declines, and their population health suffers. When involved in actual violent conflict, states are forced to address escalating population health needs with this diminished capacity. During times of war, public health needs of societies increase dramatically due to the direct casualties of war as well as the indirect negative effects of violent conflict, including widespread disease and disability. However, the resources allocated to health are lower than prewar levels, and that has serious ramifications for population well-being and health achievement.

It is important to note that, in addition to diversion of resources from welfare to warfare, states that are involved in conflict—particularly longer conflicts—experience a decrease in their overall income levels. This compounds the decline in states' capacity to provide adequate public health. According to the United Nations Children's Fund (UNICEF) estimates, by 1986 Mozambique's GDP was 50 percent less than what it would have been without the war, and Mozambique became the poorest state in the world. The number of effective health care facilities decreased due to the actual combat as well as lack of health care workers as a result of extremely low real wages. Government spending on health decreased by 40 percent in real terms between 1980 and 1991 (Noormahomed and Cliff 2002). The public health effects of the economic cost of war in Mozambique included severe disease epidemics, malnutrition, and low immunization rates. Measles, plague, meningitis, and scabies are just a few of the epidemics that spread due to the war and the state's economic inability to meet its health care needs, such as provision of sanitary living conditions and vaccinations. The decreased levels of health care provision also influenced the treatment of the direct casualties of war, drastically increasing war-mortality. The countries of West Africa—including Niger, Sierra Leone, and Liberia—have also been expanding defense spending at the cost of other sectors of the economy, particularly health and education (Raheem and Akinroye 2002). These budgetary trade-offs have been accompanied by extremely low public health outputs and a lack of basic health care services.

The level of public health in a society is largely determined by the resources—economic and human—that are allocated to the health sector. Involvement in violent conflict simultaneously forces states to increase spending on defense and increases the need for public health provision. Violent conflict also impedes the normal economic activities of a state, including disruptions in trade due to combat or sanctions. The resources available to a state are limited under any circumstances, but these resources become even more scarce during times of war. Hence states are left with a smaller pie and demands for a larger slice for military expenditures. The need for defense is pressing and, consequently, other uses are allocated fewer resources. As a result, health expenditures decrease at a time when public health demands are increasing due to the direct and indirect health effects of armed conflict. Combat results in the destruction of infrastructure, including health facilities and hospitals. Due to the destruction of war, the numbers of functioning health care facilities and personnel decrease. Not just economic resources, but health care personnel may also be diverted from civilian to military use to cope with war casualties. Thus war reduces health care infrastructure and human resources available to the population. Under these conditions, the diversion of economic resources away from the health sector is particularly detrimental. There are also fewer resources than in prewar times to run existing health care facilities and none to rebuild the ones that have been damaged or destroyed. There are fewer resources to employ health care workers, purchase supplies and medicine, offer vaccinations, and pay the overhead costs of facilities. As direct casualties of war—military and civilian—roll in, disease spreads and epidemics break out, and the decrease in resources makes it unlikely that the state will be able to meet its wartime health care obligations.

Several studies of budgetary trade-offs have examined the effect of defense spending on investment and economic growth (Domke et al. 1983; Rasler and Thompson 1988; Ward et al. 1995), and welfare spending (Russett 1969; Mintz and Huang 1991; Apostolakis 1992). These studies examine the effect of expenditures in the defense sector on various aspects of the economy, such as growth and investment. They do not, however, consider the direct effect of involvement in violent conflict on either defense expenditure or welfare spending. I assess the effect of violent conflict on the health and human security of populations by evaluating the diversion of resources from health expenditures toward defense spending. I argue that the need for increased defense spending due to involvement in conflict compels states to divert resources from human services, such as health and education, toward defense expenditures. This diversion of resources is an important mechanism through which violent conflict undermines the health of populations.

In summary, I offer two broad expectations regarding the relationships among violent conflict, defense spending, and spending on social and public health programs. First, I hypothesize that, due to war, the overall economic resources—reflected in national income—will decline. Conflict disrupts aspects of a society's economic activity and results in fewer resources. Second, I hypothesize that public health is undermined by violent conflict due to diversion of economic resources from welfare and human services to military expenditures. Thus, the already limited pool of resources available to states becomes even smaller during times of conflict, and a larger share of these reduced resources goes toward military spending. In the next section, I briefly discuss the possible effect of conflict on the national income of states and the government share of the national income. Next, I examine how states decide between defense and social spending in the presence of violent conflict.

CONFLICT AND ECONOMIC RESOURCES

Public spending decisions occur in an environment of finite resources and the level of these limited resources is affected by involvement in militarized conflict. All aspects of spending—public and private—in an economy are functions of the overall national income. Involvement in militarized conflict has a negative effect on many of the economic activities of a state and is likely to reduce national wealth and productivity. Hence, the pie that is to be divided among competing public uses—including defense and health—gets smaller as states become engaged in conflict.

Table 7.1 shows the effect of conflict on GDP, as well as the portion of the national income that is allocated to government uses. I test this relationship by estimating a regression model with country-specific fixed effects. This is not meant to be a comprehensive model of either GDP or government spending but merely presents an illustration of how conflict might affect economic resources at the broader level.[16] I control for regime type and use the POLITY IV scale as a measure of democracy. I include a lagged dependent variable to account for the effect of time. The inclusion of a lagged dependent variable eliminates the problem of serial correlation but can induce the issue of sapping the independent variables of their explanatory power (Achen 2000). I, therefore, report two sets of results, with and without a lagged dependent variable.

Table 7.1. Effect of Conflict on Economic Resources, 1970–2000

	Per-Capita GDP		Government Share of GDP	
	No Lagged Y	Lagged Y	No Lagged Y	Lagged Y
(Constant)	5.86**	0.10**	19.78**	2.48**
	(0.04)	(0.01)	(0.11)	(0.16)
Y_{it-1}	—	1.01**	—	0.87**
		(<0.01)		(0.01)
POLITY score	0.085**	−0.00	−0.04*	−0.02
	(0.01)	(<0.01)	(0.02)	(0.01)
Minor Conflict	−0.27*	−0.02	0.50	0.30
	(−2.13)	(0.02)	(0.33)	(0.16)
Major Conflict	−0.14	−0.07**	2.83**	0.73**
	(1.03)	(0.02)	(0.35)	(0.17)
R^2	0.40	0.99	0.03	0.93
N	4,492	4,346	4,507	4,358

NOTE: Cell entries are coefficient estimates; numbers in parentheses are standard errors. * = $p < .05$; ** = $p < .01$ (one-tailed).

According to this simple analysis, the national income of states is likely to decrease due to involvement in conflict, particularly major conflict. The first two columns report the results of the analysis for per-capita GDP and suggest that overall societal wealth is, as expected, negatively influenced by the presence of violent conflict. Similar results are found in the model that includes a lagged dependent variable. As hypothesized, involvement in violent conflict has a negative effect on resources. Specifically, the model in the first column suggests that annual per-capita GDP decreases by $270 due to minor conflicts.

The decrease in GDP, however, may not necessarily be dispositive, since governments might actually spend more in times of war. As the national income of states decreases due to involvement in conflict, states may apportion a larger share of the GDP for government purposes. This increase in the government slice of the national income, however, is coming out of a smaller pie. Moreover, this increase in the state share of GDP is a result of heightened security concerns and is unlikely to be spent on expenditures such as health and social welfare. It is not certain what this higher percentage of the government portion of national income means in terms of real public expenditures, particularly in the nondefense sectors. As the government takes over more of the society's resources for its war effort, further deterioration of the economy might occur due to shrinkage of the private sector. It is important to note that even in cases in which absolute spending on health remains constant during times of war, the levels of health outputs decrease due to the increased burdens placed on population health.

Therefore, involvement in conflict is negatively related to national income, and this complicates public spending decisions. As the overall level of resources declines, states apportion a larger percentage of these resources for government uses. However, this increase in government resources may not mean much in real terms due to the decrease in GDP. Moreover, government resources during periods of conflict are more likely to be used for defense purposes than for social and human services. In the next section, I examine the influence of conflict on various aspects of public expenditures and assess the existence of trade-offs between defense and health spending. Does involvement in militarized conflict induce states to increase defense spending at the expense of services such as public health? I argue that in spite of a possible increase in the government portion of the GDP, conflict results in diversion of resources from health to military spending, and I test this relationship in the model presented below.

A MODEL OF DEFENSE-WELFARE EXPENDITURES

To analyze the relationship between violent conflict and the allocation of economic resources, I use a system of equations and assess how involvement in minor or major militarized conflict influences states' spending on defense, health, and education. I evaluate the effect of conflict on defense, health, and education expenditures in 112 countries, for which these public spending data are available, from 1970 to 2000. Although government spending on education is not of central interest in this analysis, it has been included in the model because education is a major component of public spending in most countries and is generally expected to suffer due to increased defense expenditures. Including education expenditures in the models gives a clearer idea of how higher levels of military spending due to conflict affect social services and the welfare of societies. Education spending may also be viewed as a proxy for government engagement in social development and human capital.

Data and Operationalization

The dependent variables in this analysis are defense expenditures, public health expenditures, and education expenditures. The purpose of the model is to assess the trade-off between defense and health spending, but I have included education since it is a major component of social spending and is also likely to be affected by higher levels of defense spending. To measure these government expenditures, I use the Government Financial Statistics data, which have been put together by the International Monetary Fund. These data are collected yearly "primarily by means of a detailed questionnaire distributed to government financial statistics correspondents, who are usually located in each country's respective ministry of finance or central bank" (International Monetary Fund 1993) and contain statistics on government revenue, expenditures, and debt. Government expenditure is disaggregated into a number of categories, including defense, health, and education.

The variables of interest in my analysis are the proportions of all government spending devoted to defense, health, education, and other activities for each country in each year. I measure defense, health, and education expenditures as a proportion of the total central government expenditures for each year. For the country-years in these data, defense spending ranges from zero to 100 percent of total government expenditures; health spending ranges between zero to 84 percent of public spending; and education expenditures range from zero to 61 percent of total spending. These are compositional data (Aitchison 1986), with "multiple outcome variables that sum to unity for each observation" (Katz and King 1999, 19), as they deal with proportions of the total budget. To avoid assuming that the ratios of the various aspects of public spending are independent, I follow Aitchison (1986) and estimate a seemingly unrelated regression model of spending categories. That is, I model the log of the ratio of the proportion of the budget spent on defense, health, and education to that spent on other activities. So, for

Table 7.2. Summary Statistics for Defense-Welfare Model, 1970–2000

Variables	Mean	Standard Deviation	Minimum	Maximum
Dependent Variables				
Defense	−2.17	0.83	−4.98	0.01
Health	−2.60	0.92	−6.50	−0.24
Education	−1.99	0.84	−6.11	−0.58
Independent Variables				
Minor Conflict	0.14	0.35	0	1
Major Conflict	0.09	0.28	0	1
POLITY score	3.58	7.12	−10	10
Per-Capita GDP	8.54	6.96	0.28	33.29

NOTE: $N = 1,639$.

health spending, my dependent variable is:

$$Y_{Health} = ln \left[\frac{\text{Health Spending}_{it}/\text{All Spending}_{it}}{\text{Other Spending}_{it}/\text{All Spending}_{it}} \right]$$

I calculate similar ratios for defense and education spending; each is calculated relative to the residual category *Other Spending*.

The main independent variable is conflict. As in the analyses in previous chapters, I consult data from the Peace Research Institute of Oslo (PRIO) on armed conflict (Gleditsch et al. 2002), and I categorize conflict as *Major Conflict* and *Minor Conflict*.[17] I also control for democracy and wealth. The democracy variable (*POLITY score*) reflects the regime type of a state and is measured similarly to previous analyses (by its POLITY IV score). The wealth variable (*Per-Capita GDP*) is the real GDP of a state. The summary statistics for these variables, for observations that are included in the model, are shown in Table 7.2. In the next section, I present the empirical analysis of budgetary trade-offs in states that are involved in armed conflict.

Analysis and Results

I estimate the model as a system of equations through an approach referred to as Zellner's seemingly unrelated regression (SUR). This approach allows simultaneous estimation of all equations in the system and is asymptotically more efficient than single-equation least-squares estimators if the equations have contemporaneously correlated error terms (Zellner 1962).

Table 7.3. Defense, Health, and Education Spending During Conflict, 1970–2000

	Defense	Health	Education
Constant	−2.25**	−2.67**	−1.56**
	(0.03)	(0.04)	(0.03)
POLITY score	−0.05**	0.03**	< 0.01
	(< 0.01)	(< 0.01)	(< 0.01)
Per-Capita GDP	0.02**	< 0.01	−0.05**
	(< 0.01)	(< 0.01)	(< 0.01)
Minor Conflict	0.58**	−0.16*	−0.20**
	(0.05)	(0.06)	(0.06)
Major Conflict	0.57**	−0.21**	−0.10
	(0.06)	(0.08)	(0.07)
SEE	0.72	0.88	0.77
R^2	0.25	0.10	0.15
N	1,639	1,639	1,639

NOTE: Cell entries are coefficient estimates; numbers in parentheses are standard errors. * = $p < .05$; ** = $p < .01$ (one-tailed).

A SUR model is appropriate because, to the extent that the estimates are influenced by factors not included in the model, it is important to allow the error terms to be correlated. Hence, I estimate the following three equations simultaneously:

$$Defense = \beta_0 + \beta_1 Democracy + \beta_2 Minor\ Conflict + \beta_3 Major\ Conflict$$
$$+ \beta_4 GDP + \mu_d$$

$$Health = \gamma_0 + \gamma_1 Democracy + \gamma_2 Minor\ Conflict + \gamma_3 Major\ Conflict$$
$$+ \gamma_4 GDP + \mu_h$$

$$Education = \delta_0 + \delta_1 Democracy + \delta_2 Minor\ Conflict + \delta_3 Major\ Conflict$$
$$+ \delta_4 GDP + \mu_e$$

Table 7.3 shows the results for the model evaluating budgetary trade-offs between defense and welfare expenditures due to conflict. This analysis provides strong support for the hypothesis that, in times of war, states are inclined to increase their spending on defense and decrease public spending on health. Government expenditures on education also decline as wartime spending on defense rises. This reveals states' propensity to favor defense expenditures over social welfare and health when their security needs are heightened due to involvement in conflict.

States that are involved in violent conflict are likely to increase their defense expenditures by about 57 percent, and this increase is consistent across various intensities of conflict. Even states involved in minor conflict increase their defense spending to the same degree as states involved in high-intensity conflict. During 1991, Kuwait's military spending went up by 211 percent, while health expenditures decreased by 88 percent. Military expenditures are likely to go up as much during periods of preparation for war as when states are actually fighting a war; that explains steep rises in defense spending even for lower-intensity conflicts. Involvement in any conflict raises the threat level of states and compels them to strengthen their military readiness.

The heightened need for defense spending is reflected in other areas of public expenditures, such as public health. Health spending decreases by 16 percent when states are involved in minor conflict and by 21 percent due to major or high-intensity conflict. Similarly, education expenditures are likely to shrink by 20 percent due to involvement in militarized conflict. Although there are a number of other aspects of public spending—not included in this model—that are also affected by increased defense budgets to cope with military threats, there is clear evidence that resources allocated to population health are negatively influenced by these budgetary changes. At least a significant portion of the higher defense budget is at the expense of health spending, which is particularly important since war raises states' health care needs.

Democracy, as measured by states' POLITY scores, is negatively related to defense spending. Lower levels of democracy are associated with higher defense expenditures. Israel is an exception in that, despite high levels of democracy (POLITY scores of 9 or 10), the country has maintained high levels of defense spending due to unusual security threats and persistent involvement in various degrees of militarized conflict. Mintz and Ward (1989) argue that Israel's high defense expenditures may be attributed to political manipulation by the defense sector. However, Israel's defense spending has decreased significantly since the 1970s; in 1976, 42 percent of Israel's total spending was for defense, compared to 17 percent in 2001. The level of democracy is positively related to health expenditures, which is

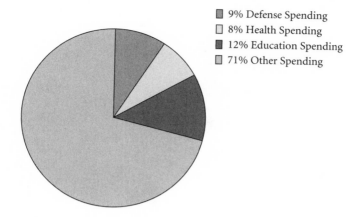

Figure 7.1. Public Expenditures in the Absence of Conflict

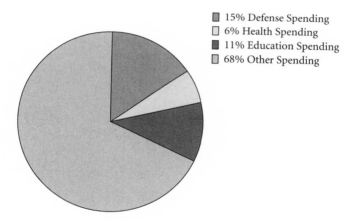

Figure 7.2. Public Expenditures in the Presence of Minor Conflict

consistent with the arguments that democracies invest more in human capital than nondemocratic states do (Baum and Lake 2003). National income is positively related to defense spending and has no significant effect on health expenditures.

Figures 7.1, 7.2, 7.3, and 7.4 illustrate the effect of conflict on governments' budgetary decisions. In the absence of any armed conflict, an average state in the system during the time considered (with a per-capita GDP of $8,600 and a defense expenditure of 8.6 percent), spent 9 percent of its

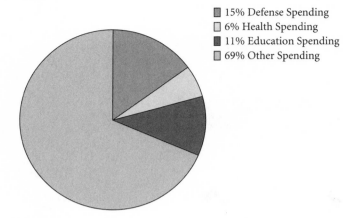

15% Defense Spending
6% Health Spending
11% Education Spending
69% Other Spending

Figure 7.3. Public Expenditures in the Presence of Major Conflict (totals exceed 100 percent due to rounding)

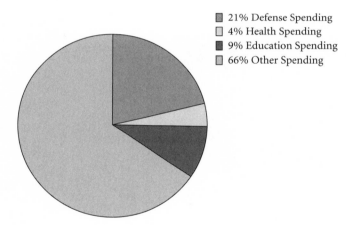

21% Defense Spending
4% Health Spending
9% Education Spending
66% Other Spending

Figure 7.4. Public Expenditures in the Presence of Both Minor and Major Conflict

entire government expenditure on defense, 8 percent on health, and 12 percent on education (see Figure 7.1). With involvement in either minor or major conflict, the spending on defense went up to 15 percent, while health and education expenditures declined to 6 and 11 percent, respectively (see Figures 7.2 and 7.3). For states that were involved in both high-intensity and minor conflicts, the trade-offs were the most profound. These states increased their defense expenditures to 21 percent, decreased their education spending to 9 percent, and reduced spending on health to 6 percent (see Figure 7.4).

CONCLUSION

The analysis in this chapter clearly demonstrates that involvement in conflict is likely to induce state governments to divert resources from social uses, including health and education, toward defense expenditures. The propensity of states to favor defense spending over health expenditures reflects adherence to traditional notions of security that focus on military power. These budgetary trade-offs, however, have significant consequences for human security as the higher defense budgets emerge at the cost of public expenditures that are crucial to overall social development. Education, social security, public housing, welfare programs, and investment are all important elements of development and human security. And all these factors are negatively affected by increases in defense spending, with repercussions for development and economic growth. However, the diversion of resources from health expenditures in times of conflict reflects the most significant threat to human security. Health is the core component of human security, without which other elements of security—such as economic prosperity and environmental safety—cannot fully be enjoyed.

During conflict, the health of populations is negatively impacted from two directions. War results in higher rates of mortality, injury, disability, and disease. The immediate and delayed effects of combat leave populations with serious health concerns that call for mobilization of extra resources to meet these health needs. Instead, states tend to reduce resources allocated to health, leaving many of the population's health needs unmet. Even if states manage to maintain absolute expenditures on health during times of war, the health achievement of society may still decline due to the extra health burden resulting from conflict. In order to maintain prewar levels of population health, it may be necessary to significantly increase the level of resources allocated to both preventive and curative health. The analysis here has only looked at economic resources, but it should be noted that human resources—including health care personnel—are also diverted from civilian to military uses during conflict. That puts further strain on the civilian populations. The effects of war on public health due to economic constraints are obvious in many conflict-ridden states, particularly in Africa.

In this chapter, I have discussed the diversion of economic resources from health to defense as an important mechanism through which militarized conflict negatively influences the ability of states to provide adequate health care to their populations. In the next chapter, I examine the effect of forced migration on health outcomes in states that host large refugee groups.

8

FORCED MIGRATION
AND POPULATION HEALTH

AS DEMONSTRATED IN PREVIOUS CHAPTERS, the indirect effects of violent conflict on population health occur through a number of mechanisms. The last chapter examined the relationship between war and the diversion of economic resources from social to defense spending. In this chapter, I examine the effect of conflict on public health through forced migration and the generation of refugee flows. Both civil and interstate conflicts are often associated with displacement of groups of people, who either remain displaced within their own state or cross national borders to enter another state for safe haven. The implications of forced migration for human security are highly significant and multifaceted. People who are forced to leave their homes due to the exigencies of war are confronted with a host of threats to their security, ranging from the circumstances that compelled them to migrate to protracted insecure conditions in the host country. On the other side, the receiving state may not be adequately equipped to deal with the needs of the refugee population without considerable strain on its society and resources, hence threatening the security of the host population as well.

Since the focus of this book is to examine the health effects of war at the national or population level, I evaluate the impact that the influx of refugee groups has on societal health levels in states to which they migrate. This linkage in the war-and-health relationship is different from other linkages that I have examined because the effect of forced migration occurs in a country other than the one in which the war takes place. This effect of war on health reflects the dispersion of the consequences of armed conflict and thus highlights the global nature of this issue. I argue that refugee populations that are produced by violent conflict migrate to states with lower levels of conflict; after their migration to those states, the target states experience a deterioration in their health outcomes. Below I briefly discuss the nature of conflict-induced forced migration in the current international system, followed by my expectations for the effect of forced migration on public health, and then I present an empirical analysis of this relationship for the period from 1965 to 1995.

FORCED MIGRATION AS A SECURITY ISSUE

The United Nations defines refugees as "people who are outside their countries because of a well-founded fear of persecution . . . and cannot or do not want to return home" (United Nations High Commissioner for Refugees 2005, 5). The end of the Cold War saw a surge of ethnic conflict and secessionist movements that resulted in displacement and migration of large groups of people. Although a number of those conflicts have been resolved—such as the ones in former Yugoslavia—civil wars remain a major source of refugee flows in Africa. In his discussion of the causes of forced migration, Posen (1996) lists a number of factors that are directly associated with violent conflict. For instance, "politicide" against proponents of certain beliefs, genocide of enemy groups, and ethnic cleansings to achieve homogeneity are among the chief determinants of forced migration. Moreover, people may flee their homes for fear of being caught in the violence of combat, of being the victims of "primitive logistics" whereby combat forces raid local communities for resources, or to avoid occupation by the opposing side. For instance, most of the Chechen population left the city of Grozny before the Russians arrived to avoid the potential dangers of being trapped in a combat zone (Posen 1996). Whether people become displaced due to deliberate evacuations by enemy forces or due to the dangerous conditions fostered by armed conflict, they generally depart in desperate conditions and are exposed to a range of human security threats. Clearly the migrant group is not secure; their physical, mental, and economic well-being is severely affected and the prospects for their future are uncertain. But forced migration also presents salient threats to the security of the state that receives the refugees as it grapples with the issues of accommodating the newcomers.[18]

During the Cold War years, most of the refugee migration occurred from the communist Eastern Bloc to the democratic states of the West due to political repression. Refugees generally left their home countries as individuals or in small groups, and those who managed to circumvent the stringent exit restrictions of their home countries were encouraged and assisted by the receiving countries (Iqbal and Zorn 2007).[19] After the Cold War, the nature of refugee flows and international response to it changed as violent conflicts resulted in large-scale migration of people who escaped dangerous situations in desperate conditions. For example, the war in Rwanda alone created 2.5 million refugees. The international community rapidly became aware of the destabilizing effects of such large-scale movement of people and international organizations, as well as refugee recipient states, began to discourage forced migration and to create solutions to the global refugee issue. For instance, the United Nations High Commissioner for Refugees (UNHCR) works actively to create adequate conditions for repatriation of refugees—including technical, financial, and transportation assistance (United Nations High Commissioner for Refugees 2005).

Of key concern to the international community are protracted forced displacement situations, where both the refugee and host populations experience long-term challenges to their security. Resolutions to refugee situations include settlement into the host state, resettlement in a third state, and repatriation to the home state under safe conditions. The UNHCR's *State of the World's Refugees* (2006) presents a mixed picture of the global refugee crisis:

> International efforts to improve refugee assistance and protection have been aided in recent years by the easing of some of the acute displacement crises that dominated the 1990s. Furthermore, there have been breakthroughs in the resolution of a number of long-running conflicts, allowing many refugees to return to their countries of

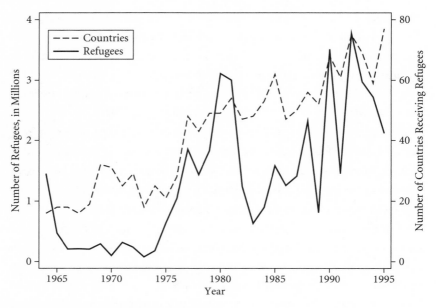

Figure 8.1. Trends in Refugee Flows, 1965–1995

origin. The global population of refugees of concern to UNHCR has declined in recent years, from nearly 18 million in 1992 to just over 9 million in 2004. This is mainly due to a drop in the number of armed conflicts and several large-scale repatriations. But despite the reduction in the total number of refugees worldwide, the majority of those who remain live without any prospect of a durable solution to their plight. In 2004, there were some 33 situations of protracted refugee exile involving 5.7 million refugees. (10)

The efforts by the international community to repatriate refugees reflect the recognition of the security threats posed to the receiving states by these situations, both in the form of effects on the domestic population and on the immigrant group. Given the conditions under which most refugees escape their home states, their destination choices are often quite limited and they tend to migrate to neighboring and nearby states (Iqbal 2007). Forced migration can, therefore, lead to instability in neighboring states or an entire region and thus represents a particularly salient consequence of conflict. Figure 8.1 shows the trends in refugee flows over the period from

1965 to 1995. In the next section, I outline the relationships among violent conflict, refugee flows, and population health.

WAR, REFUGEES, AND HEALTH

Most interstate migration occurs due to economic reasons as people leave their countries in search of better opportunities. Refugees, however, are not economic migrants and enter another state to escape persecution or physical danger. Reports by international agencies such as UNHCR as well as academic research provide ample evidence that violence in the home state is the most important determinant of forced migration. Davenport et al. (2003) assess the dynamics of forced migration during the period from 1964 to 1989 and find that violent state and dissident behavior is the chief cause for people to become migrants; civil wars, genocides, and politicides are of particular importance in the creation of refugee flows. In a similar study of the determinants of forced migration during the period from 1952 to 1995, Moore and Shellman (2004) also find that violence in a state—both by the government and dissidents—has a much greater impact on levels of forced migration than other socioeconomic factors, such as the type of regime and national income. The large-scale refugee flows created by armed conflicts, such as the ones in the former Yugoslavia and the Soviet invasion of Afghanistan, demonstrate the staggering impact of war on populations through mass displacement. Civil wars in sub-Saharan Africa have also been associated with massive refugee flows: for example, the domestic conflicts in Rwanda, Liberia, Somalia, and the Sudan.

War and other forms of violence in their home states are indeed the main reason people decide to become refugees. However, people also have to decide on a state to which to migrate. In addition to examining the determinants of forced migration, some studies have focused on the characteristics of states targeted by refugees as their destination. Intuition suggests that refugees would flee to a country in which conditions—particularly with respect to violence—are better than in their home states. Moore and Shellman (2007) assess the characteristics of refugee receiving states during the period from 1965 to 1995 and find that among the influences on refugee inflows are contiguity and colonial ties. Their analysis suggests an increase in the likelihood of civil war in a state that hosts refugees; they also find that refugees tend to migrate to states that have previously received refugees. Weiner (1996) also contends that refugee flows are associated with regional instability and occur most prominently in "violence-prone bad neighborhoods." According to Iqbal (2007), however, the most significant determining factor in refugee destinations is distance; refugees are most likely to migrate to states that they can reach easily given that they generally do not have access to adequate transportation. Consequently, refugee groups migrate to neighboring and nearby states, and the effects of other factors in the receiving states—such as levels of democracy—are mediated by the distance between the home and target states.

Here I argue that refugees' choice of destination is likely to be influenced more by their ability to reach a state that does not have the same levels of violence and conflict than by a state's socioeconomic capacity to accommodate and cater to the needs of the migrant group. This implies that inflows of refugees can be destabilizing for host states, including an impact on their health achievements. Particularly, in light of the findings of Moore and Shellman (2007), refugees are likely to seek shelter in states that have received refugees in the past, which could exacerbate the destabilizing effects of refugee inflows. Weiner (1992) provides an extensive discussion of the possible security threats caused by large-scale migration. These threats, he argues, include threats to cultural identity, political consequences for the relationship with the refugees' home country, and socioeconomic burden.[20] With respect to the social and economic strain caused by refugee inflows, Weiner (1992) states:

> Societies may react to immigrants because of the economic costs they impose or because of their purported social behavior such as criminality, welfare dependency, delinquency, etc. Societies may be concerned because the people entering are so numerous or so poor that they create a substantial economic burden by straining housing, education, and transportation facilities. (114)

Large refugee flows can also strain the health care systems of host states, thereby inhibiting the ability of societies to maintain or improve their health outcome levels. Refugees escape war and violence in their home states and are likely to be injured or in ill health when they arrive at their destination. Moreover, refugee groups often live under conditions that are associated with proliferation of disease, such as crowded camps and widespread malnutrition.[21] These groups are thus likely to have higher health care needs and, in addition to adding to the number of people whose health care needs have to be met by the host state, they may increase the incidence of certain diseases in the receiving society through contagion.[22]

Large-scale refugee flows, therefore, disperse the health effects of violent conflict in their home states to the countries to which they migrate. As previous chapters have demonstrated, incidence of violent conflict is associated with lower health outcomes and war affects health in both direct and indirect ways, such as through infrastructural damage and resource diversion. The impact of refugee flows on health, however, occurs in the state that receives the refugees and thus reflects the diffusion of the effects of war. In this chapter, I evaluate the relationships among war, refugee inflows, and public health. I argue that armed conflict compels groups of people to leave their homes and these refugees seek shelter in states that do not have the same levels of violence. The arrival of these refugees results in a negative impact on the health outputs in the state that receives them due to the low levels of health achievement among the migrant groups and the burden placed on the host state's health care apparatus. Hence, the effect of violent conflict on health through forced migration occurs in a state that is not involved in conflict.

Since refugees are likely to migrate to states without or with lower levels of conflict, one would not expect to find a strong bivariate correlation between forced migration and health achievement. Figure 8.2 reflects the lack of a bivariate correlation between levels of refugee flows into a state and its infant mortality rates;[23] similar bivariate effects exist between refugee flows and fertility rates and life expectancy. The reason for the absence of a linear relationship between forced migration and indicators of public health is that refugees migrate to states with lower levels of conflict and higher levels of health outputs than their home countries. As a result, given that conflict reduces health levels, states with conflict will have health

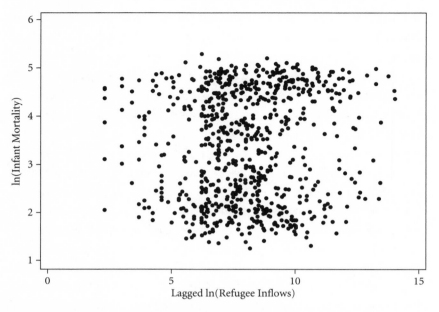

Figure 8.2. Bivariate Relationship Between Refugee Inflows and Infant Mortality, 1965–1995

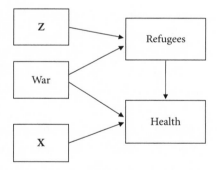

Figure 8.3. War, Refugees, and Health

achievement levels that are not much different from health outcomes in states that do not have conflict but harbor large numbers of refugees. Figure 8.3 conceptualizes the linkages among refugee inflows, war in the recipient state, and health in the host state; Z and X represent other exogenous factors that influence both health and refugee flows. I argue that war in the host country decreases refugee flows, and refugee flows decrease health outputs. The best way to assess the endogenous relationships among conflict, forced migration, and health is through an instrumental variables approach similar to the one adopted in Chapter 6 to evaluate the linkages among war, infrastructure, and public health. Here, this approach allows me to examine how conflict affects health in states other than the one that creates the refugee flows. I am thus able to examine the neighborhood or regional effects of war on health as the impact of war diffuses across borders through migration. Below I present the data and the empirical analysis of the war-refugees-health relationship during the period from 1965 to 1995.

DATA AND OPERATIONALIZATION

I evaluate the effect of refugee inflows on population health in all country-years from 1965 to 1995. The dependent variables in this analysis are *Life Expectancy*, *Infant Mortality*, and *Fertility Rates*; these indicators measure public health at the national level. The data for these variables were obtained from the *World Development Indicators* (World Bank 2006), and they are operationalized in a similar manner as in the analyses in Chapters 5 and 6. Life expectancy denotes the average number of years an individual in a population is expected to live and ranges from 31.22 (Cambodia in 1977) to 79.70 years (Japan in 1994) in the sample. Infant mortality rates reflect the number of infant deaths per 1,000 live births in a population (the variable is logged), and fertility rates measure the average number of children to whom women in a population give birth. Higher levels of life expectancy and lower levels of fertility and infant mortality reflect higher health achievement.

The main independent variable in this analysis is the number of refugees that enter a state in a given year. I use the Moore and Shellman (1997) data set for measuring refugee flows. Moore and Shellman (1997) employ the annual estimated stock of refugees in a country provided by UNHCR to calculate annual flows by taking the first difference in the stock and then truncating it at zero to avoid negative values.[24] It should be noted that refugee flows are a rare event and for most of the country-years in the sample, the refugee inflows were zero. Among the country-years with positive refugee flows, the number of refugees ranged from 10 to more than 1.3 million. The *Refugee Flows* variable is logged in the analysis. I expect refugee stock in a state to

Table 8.1. Summary Statistics

Variables	Observations	Mean	Standard Deviation	Minimum	Maximum
Dependent Variables					
Life Expectancy	2,741	60.89	11.98	31.22	79.70
ln(Infant Mortality)	3,308	3.66	1.01	1.16	5.57
Fertility Rates	3,345	4.06	2.05	1.17	10.13
Independent Variables					
Lagged ln(Refugee Flows)	5,123	2.06	3.72	0	14.10
Lagged Major Conflict	6,475	0.07	0.27	0	1
Lagged Minor Conflict	6,475	0.08	0.27	0	1
Lagged POLITY score	4,824	−0.94	7.57	−10	10
Lagged ln(Per-Capita GDP)	4,390	7.46	1.52	4.34	10.77
Lagged ln(Trade Openness)	4,288	4.01	0.65	1.23	6.08
Lagged ln(Population)	6,203	15.26	1.91	10.63	20.90
Year (1960 = 0)	7,395	17.61	10.33	0	35

have a positive effect on both fertility and infant mortality rates and to cause a decrease in life expectancy.

Two measures of conflict are included in the model, major and minor conflict.[25] Note that these variables are indicators of conflict in the state to which refugees migrate and I expect conflict to have a negative influence on the three measures of population health, which is to say that the presence of armed conflict will decrease life expectancy and increase fertility and infant mortality rates. I control for the effects of democracy, national income, economic openness, and population.[26] The *POLITY Score, Per-Capita GDP, Trade Openness,* and *Population* variables have been lagged. Consistent with arguments presented in the previous chapters, I expect democracy, wealth, and population to improve the three health outcomes in the model. I also expect the three indicators of public health to improve over time and, therefore, have included a variable for year, with 1960 being zero. Except *Year,* all independent variables have been lagged by one year to account for the effect of time. Summary statistics are presented in Table 8.1.

ANALYSIS AND RESULTS

I analyze the effect of conflict-generated refugee flows on population health in the host country through an instrumental variables approach, using a two-stage least squares model. I employed a similar model in Chapter 6 to evaluate the effect of conflict on resource allocation in public spending. In the analysis in this chapter, the instrumental variables approach requires at least one variable that affects refugee flows but does not influence health outputs. Therefore, in the first stage of the analysis, I use refugee flows lagged two years ($Refugee\ Inflows_{t-2}$) to instrument the main independent variable of refugee flows lagged one year. The one-period lag in the independent variable accounts for the expectation that the impact of refugee flows on health would occur at a lag. Refugee flows at a two-period lag is a factor that is plausibly related to refugee flows at a one-year lag but not an influence on current health levels. It has been shown in existing literature (e.g., Moore and Shellman 2007) that refugees migrate to states to which previous refugee flows have occurred; new refugees know that these states allow refugee inflows and possibly have ties to the existing refugees. It has also been established that most refugees migrate to nearby states (e.g., Iqbal 2007), which suggests that these states would continue to receive refugees from prolonged conflicts. Therefore, refugee flows two years ago have a direct effect on refugee flows at time $t - 1$. However, refugee flows at $t - 2$ have no direct effect on health outcomes; their effect on health only occurs indirectly through refugee flows at $t - 1$.

The results of the statistical model, presented in Table 8.2 reveal a significantly detrimental effect of forced migration into a state on the three indicators of public health.[27] I find that a 1 percent increase in refugee flows decreases life expectancy by about four months, increases fertility rates by 0.1, and raises infant mortality rates by 2 percent. These findings provide evidence for the hypotheses outlined above regarding the effect of refugee flows into a country on its population health and demonstrate that hosting large migrant groups does, indeed, take a toll on a society's well-being. I have already established in previous analyses that armed conflict has direct and indirect effects on health levels in the states that are involved in conflicts. Here I show that forced migration is a significant mechanism through which conflict reduces population health in other states and can, therefore, lead to widespread regional health ramifications. These sorts of regional dynamics are apparent in sub-Saharan Africa, where civil wars have forced masses

Table 8.2. Refugee Flows and Public Health, 1965–1995

Variables	Life Expectancy	Fertility Rates	Infant Mortality
Constant	−5.66	17.50	9.76
	(30.3)	(0.53)	(0.2)
Lagged ln(Refugee Flows)	−0.36**	0.10**	0.02**
	(0.08)	(0.01)	(0.005)
Lagged Major Conflict	−0.85	0.42**	0.18**
	(0.69)	(0.12)	(0.05)
Lagged Minor Conflict	−0.24	−0.07	−0.01
	(0.60)	(1.11)	(0.04)
Lagged POLITY score	0.24**	−0.07**	−0.02**
	(0.02)	(0.004)	(−0.002)
Lagged ln(Per-Capita GDP)	5.06**	−0.72**	−0.48**
	(0.12)	(0.02)	(0.01)
Lagged ln(Trade Openness)	1.11**	−0.36**	−0.14**
	(0.33)	(0.06)	(0.02)
Lagged ln(Population)	1.23**	−0.34**	−0.08**
	(0.13)	(0.02)	(0.01)
Year (1960 = 0)	0.26**	−0.05**	−0.03**
	(0.02)	(0.003)	(0.001)
R^2	0.77	0.72	0.85
N	1,458	1,867	1,891

NOTE: Cell entries are two-stage least squares coefficient estimates; robust standard errors clustered by country are in parentheses. * = $p < .05$; ** = $p < .01$ (one-tailed).

of refugees to migrate to neighboring states. Conflicts such as the ones in Sierra Leone, the Sudan, Liberia, Ethiopia, and Rwanda have resulted in such large-scale migration, with resultant repercussions for the entire region.

With respect to the effects of the conflict variables, the model reveals a significant effect of major conflict on fertility rates and infant mortality rates. The presence of intense conflict is associated with a 0.42 unit increase in fertility rates, which reflects a deterioration in public health. Similarly, the incidence of major conflict in a country-year leads to an 18 percent increase in infant mortality rates. The effect of major conflict on life expectancy is in the hypothesized direction but is not statistically significant. Minor conflict does not have a significant effect on any measure of public health. Note that this is the direct effect of conflict on health in the state that is receiving the refugees and confirms the broader expectations of this study regarding the relationship between war and health.

I find statistically significant results in the hypothesized direction for all of the control variables. Higher levels of democracy, national income, economic openness, and population are associated with higher life expectancy and lower fertility and infant mortality rates. A one-unit increase in a state's POLITY score leads to approximately a three-month increase in life expectancy, a 0.07 unit decrease in fertility rates, and a 2 percent increase in infant mortality. These findings are consistent with arguments presented elsewhere in this book as well as in other works about higher levels of concern in democratic states with societal well-being. Similarly, both GDP and openness have a positive effect on life expectancy and a negative effect on fertility and infant mortality, which reflects that wealthier states and states that trade more enjoy high levels of health outputs. The results also suggest that as population increases, life expectancy goes up and the other two indicators decline. Last, as expected, I find that health levels improve with time, as demonstrated by the coefficients for the variable for year. Specifically, a one-year increase leads to about a three-month increase in life expectancy, a 0.05 decrease in fertility, and a 3 percent decrease in infant mortality.

CONCLUSION

The analysis in this chapter demonstrates an important linkage in the war-and-health relationship by evaluating the indirect effect of conflict on public health through refugee flows. The findings of the empirical model confirm the deteriorating impact of forced migration on key indicators of population health and exhibit a positive effect of democracy, national income, and economic openness on health achievement. As armed conflict creates conditions that compel people to leave their home states, or groups are forcefully evacuated, large numbers of people flee to states that they can reach—commonly, neighboring or close-by states. Consequently, the host states have to deal with the influx of groups that have escaped their homes without any resources and are often in poor health due to the travails of war. Thus the health effects of forced migration occur, not in the country that the refugees exit, but in the state that they enter and, therefore, cause a dispersion of the negative consequences of war at the regional level.

Given the implications of forced migration for diffusion of the effects of war, a useful focus for future research would be to identify and analyze specific spatial dynamics, such as clustering, in refugee flows and related issues.

It has already been established that distance between the home and host states is a significant influence on migration decisions of refugees; further explorations of the role of geography and spatial factors in the causes and consequences of mass migration would provide valuable insights into this pressing global issue. The importance of geography and the regional effects of refugee movements are of particular concern in Africa, where millions of refugees created by violent conflicts migrate to other states within close proximity of their home country. The most worrisome refugee crises are those of protracted situations, in which refugees are "warehoused" in camps or remain displaced for extending periods of time. Although the international community has made commendable efforts to ameliorate refugee crises, "more than 60 percent of today's refugees are trapped in situations far from the international spotlight. Often characterized by long periods of exile—stretching to decades for some groups—these situations occur on most continents in . . . camps, rural settlements and urban centres. The vast majority are to be found in the world's poorest and most unstable regions" (United Nations High Commissioner for Refugees 2006, 105). Such protracted situations include refugees from Afghanistan in Iran and Pakistan, Azerbaijanian refugees in Armenia, migrants from Burundi in Tanzania, and Angolans in the Democratic Republic of Congo. Refugees from the Sudan have been in protracted situations of at least five years in Ethiopia, the Democratic Republic of Congo, Uganda, and Kenya. These examples show a pattern of migration within regions, which emphasizes the importance of refugee flows and protracted situations for regional stability and prosperity. In 2004, UNHCR (2006) identified 33 protracted refugee situations, 17 of which were in sub-Saharan Africa.

An important influence on issues related to forced migration is the intervention of international institutions and nongovernmental organizations. Iqbal and Zorn (2007) demonstrate that the effect of civil wars on refugee creation has declined since the end of the Cold War and attribute the diminished impact of internal conflict on forced migration to interventions by global and regional organizations. Through the efforts of UNHCR and other international agencies, large-scale repatriations and resettlements have occurred since 1990 in Africa and Asia, including repatriation of large numbers of Mozambicans and Namibians and settlement of Laotian and Vietnamese refugees in third countries (United Nations High Commissioner for Refugees 2006). International efforts thus mediate the effect of conflict on migration as well as the impact of mass migration on elements of human security.

9

CONCLUSION

THE TRADITIONAL NOTIONS OF NATIONAL SECURITY focus on the security of states and their ability to guard their sovereignty against external invasion. Extended to the international level, this view of security implies that the world community is secure if its individual members—states—can protect their borders and national interests. But evolving threats to security have forced us to reevaluate this narrow, state-centric view of international security. In addition to the absence of interstate war, global security entails adequate population health, protection from environmental hazards, human rights, and social development. The concept of *human security* considers these and other elements in assessing the security of states as well as the people within states. This holistic approach to security goes beyond protection of sovereign states and their institutions and extends the idea of security to the individual level. Human security can only be achieved if communities and their individual members enjoy physical, economic, and political freedom and security. By shifting the focus of security concerns from the state to the population, this approach emphasizes the role of multiple actors in strengthening global security. States can safeguard their borders and interests, but a number of non-state actors must also be involved to achieve the security of populations. Some important non-state actors in this view of security are international organizations, nongovernmental organizations, local communities, and individuals.

At the core of human security is the physical well-being of individuals. It is through the well-being of individuals that communities, societies, and therefore, the world, can become secure. At the center of the traditional idea of security, on the other hand, is the occurrence of militarized conflict. Whereas most studies of international conflict focus on determinants of war, in this book I have examined some important aspects of the relationship between armed conflict and the health of societies. Human security is not necessarily achieved at the termination of war, and the individual elements of human security—such as health—must be studied to ascertain the security of populations. In this concluding chapter, I revisit the question of why the relationship between war and health matters to students of international security. In the next section, I briefly discuss the importance of public health as a security issue of global dimensions, followed by a discussion of some significant influences in the conflict-health relationship that might be useful directions for future research.

HEALTH AS A GLOBAL ISSUE

Is public health an issue of global security? Are threats to health a considerable security challenge? Does a focus on global health unnecessarily detract from more pressing security threats? These are questions one would expect critics of human security—or those wedded to conventional definitions of national and international security—to raise. I argue that the changing international landscape requires a broader perception of security that pays appropriate attention to various aspects of population security—including health, development, poverty, civil and human rights, and the environment. A number of disciplines have extensively studied the individual elements of human security and the salience of those issues remains unchallenged. The skepticism, however, emerges when issues such as public health are presented as threats to global security.

As Boutros-Ghali (1992) pointed out, "drought and disease can decimate no less mercilessly than the weapons of war" (2). The undeniable linkages among some major health issues and violent conflict confirm the need for focusing on the war-health relationship. These issues include the alarming rates of HIV/AIDS in sub-Saharan Africa, outbreaks of infectious diseases in refugee camps and among soldiers, and the threat of biological weapons.

Not all health issues lead to global insecurity, but a number of public health problems cannot be contained within national borders and can rapidly spread to neighboring—or even distant—states. The fear generated in the global community by Iraq's use of biological weapons against the Kurds, and the anthrax scare following September 11, 2001, manifest the extent to which acts of war can cause health threats that transcend national borders.

The Threat of Infectious Disease

The spread of infectious diseases poses as significant a threat to global security as armed conflict does. In most wars, more soldiers and civilians die of infectious diseases than actual combat. For instance, during the U.S. Civil War, twice as many soldiers died of disease as due to the fighting (McPherson 1988), and the influenza outbreak during World War I killed millions of people across Europe and other parts of the world. Even in recent conflicts, disease is often a worse killer than combat. In Liberia and Sierra Leone, diseases such as malaria and cholera have caused large numbers of deaths among troops, civilians, and peacekeepers. In 1999, it was estimated that the HIV prevalence rate in the military was up to 20 percent in Nigeria, up to 30 percent in Tanzania, and between 40 and 60 percent in Angola (Elbe 2003). Infectious diseases and other health issues are particularly harrowing due to the globalization of disease proliferation. Global interconnectedness through travel, trade, and military interventions makes it impossible to contain any health threat within a single state. It is much easier to stop militaries at borders than it is to stop viruses.

The SARS outbreak is supposed to have started in China toward the end of 2002; by early 2003, public health officials were frantically fighting the spread of the virus in Frankfurt and Toronto. Within a few months, several hundred deaths and thousands of infections had occurred as the disease diffused across several countries. The speed at which this virus travelled was a sobering awakening for governments and health practitioners across the world. But the manner in which the spread of the virus was curtailed through global cooperation and vigilance also demonstrated how health challenges can effectively be addressed only at the global level. There are "no impregnable walls between the world that is healthy, well-fed, and well-off, and another world that is sick, malnourished, and impoverished" (Brundtland 2003, 7). The merits and problems of globalization are subjected to incessant debate, and one of the effects of globalization is that health issues cannot be isolated within states or regions. Globalization, however, also facilitates the mechanisms of international cooperation that are required to mitigate and control rising health threats. Brundtland (2003) describes HIV/AIDS, tuberculosis, and malaria as the three most crucial global health threats. She estimates that more than 90 million healthy life years are lost to HIV/AIDS each year, 40 million to malaria, and 36 million to tuberculosis. Although these diseases have higher prevalence in some regions—predominantly Africa—they constitute a global burden of disease.

Disease, malnutrition, deaths, and disability in distant states are not merely relevant in that the conditions might spread across borders. Sustained levels of inadequate health outputs at the national level can lead to deteriorating economies, which in a globalized system can have far-reaching effects on the world economy. For instance, high rates of HIV/AIDS have resulted in a host of social, economic, and political problems in sub-Saharan Africa (Elbe 2002). Disease, deprivation, and the breakdown of health care in one country or region can have a global impact through devastation of markets and investments. Many consider the causal arrows between poverty and disease to be unclear or bidirectional; either way, the effect can be detrimental across the world. The significance of population health for sustainable development and growth makes it a highly salient issue in economic globalization. Globalization emphasizes the importance of a variety of actors, such as international organizations and multinational corporations; similarly, global health issues call for the involvement of state as well as non-state actors.

Health as a Human Right

Since the proclamation of the Universal Declaration of Human Rights in 1948, there has been a growing awareness of human rights as an international issue. More recently, the right to health has increasingly been brought to the fore. The notion of health as a human right started developing as global attention turned to the issue of HIV/AIDS and the large number of people living with the virus (Gruskin and Tarantola 2005). Although definitions of human rights generally apply to the relationship between individuals and the state, and how the state can or cannot treat its citizens, it is widely accepted that many issues of human rights are best addressed at the global level. A number of international organizations, led by the United Nations, have been pursuing active agendas for universal human rights for several decades. The Universal Declaration of Human Rights (UDHR) states that "everyone has the right to a standard of living adequate for the health and well-being of himself and of his family, including food, clothing, housing and medical care" (United Nations 1948). Although the UDHR includes a number of economic, social, and cultural rights, including health, the international community focused primarily on civil and political rights during the Cold War (Steiner and Alston 1996). Since the end of the Cold War, more attention has been paid to the human right to health, as outlined in the Constitution of the World Health Organization (WHO), and consisting of a "state of complete physical, mental, and social well-being" (United Nations 1946, 2).

Gruskin and Tarantola (2005) describe three specific human rights as being highly relevant to the right to health. First, the principle of nondiscrimination entails that everyone be granted the same right regardless of differences in gender, race, religion, or sexual orientation. This right applies to health in that all people and persons, by virtue of being human, have the right to achieve adequate levels of health and well-being. Also, nondiscrimination applies to the treatment of people with health conditions such as HIV/AIDS. Second, the right to the benefit of scientific progress requires that all individuals have access to medical technology and health care. The relevance of this right to public health is clear in the issue of accessibility to medication—particularly HIV/AIDS drugs—in developing countries. Although health care and technology have been improving worldwide, the distribution of the benefits of science shows significant inequalities among regions and states, as well as within states. The third is the right to health, which entails physical and mental well-being through adequate health care provision.

Acknowledging health as a human right implies that national governments and international non-state actors are bound to facilitate the provision of appropriate health and medical care to populations. Access to medical technology, facilities, and personnel is a right of each member of society, rather than a privilege reserved for a select few. Extended to the international level, the global community at large bears some responsibility for ensuring adequate health conditions around the world. This is particularly important given the prodigious inequalities in health achievement among regions, states, and within countries. In addition to health provision, viewing health as a human right reflects the necessity of creating conditions that are conducive to population well-being—including income equality within and across societies—and preventing conditions that might lead to a deterioration in public health, such as armed conflict. War undermines health and, therefore, may result in circumstances that violate a human right. The main purpose of studying the health effects of war is to elucidate the human cost of conflict and thus reduce the expected utility of waging war, thereby making war a less attractive mechanism for resolving disputes than nonviolent means. The connection between armed conflict and the human right of health also emphasizes the obligations of the international community to prevent, resolve, and intervene in violent conflicts.

VIOLENT CONFLICT AND POPULATION WELL-BEING

In this study, I have evaluated certain aspects of the relationship between conflict and health within the human security framework. I have presented public health as an international issue for which responsibility must be borne at the global level. War affects the health of societies through a host of complex mechanisms, and a number of direct and indirect consequences of violent conflict can lead to deterioration of public health. My analyses demonstrate important linkages among conflict, key sociopolitical factors, and health indicators. I find that conflict impacts the overall health of populations more severely in the short term than in the long run, that the effect of war on health varies across world regions, that democracy and wealth are positive influences on health, and that states tend to divert economic resources from health to defense due to involvement in conflict.

The implications of these findings suggest that national governments and international actors have incentives to work toward conflict prevention in order to avoid the human cost of war beyond combat. These analyses also imply that democracy is likely to lead to a healthier population and better human capital. In addition to democracy, economic resources are crucial to higher levels of health, and these resources may be taken away from health expenditures in preparation for—or during involvement in—violent conflict.

These are important conclusions regarding a significant consequence of war and are relevant to policy decisions about conflict initiation, intervention, and resource allocation. One important influence on the health impact of war that has not been empirically tested in this study, but warrants a brief discussion here, is generalized social decline that societies may experience as a result of involvement in protracted conflicts. Public health does not exist in isolation from other elements of society. Just as destruction of the general infrastructure of a society impairs its ability to provide adequate health care, the social decline that often results from involvement in conflict severely reduces the level of public health. The economic, political, and social costs imposed on a society due to conflict may result in deterioration—or even collapse—of domestic law and order, hinging on the level of devastation from, and the duration of, the conflict. Decline in domestic law and order could have similar effects on public health as the destruction of elements of infrastructure, such as transportation and communication. As law and order become less effective, the population's access to health care diminishes. Health care facilities may be located in areas that are not considered safe for either those seeking health care or health care providers. Deterioration of law and order is merely one aspect of social decline. General social decline is not a phenomenon that can easily be measured. However, it may be argued that war leads to a decline in law and order with a subsequent decline in public health outcomes. This decline in law and order may be manifested by an increase in crime rates, proliferation of violence in society, and decreased effectiveness of law-enforcement agencies. Moreover, conflict often results in a reduction of wealth in the economy, leading to the impoverishment of large segments of society and heightened inequalities of wealth and income.

Several public health scholars have argued that inequalities in income and wealth have a detrimental effect on public health in a society (Wilkinson 1996; Kawachi et al. 1997; Shi 2002).

DIRECTIONS FOR FUTURE RESEARCH

The growing international interest in issues of human security, the perpetuation of violent conflict around the world, and the analyses in this book strongly reflect the need for continued research on the relationship between war and public health. I alluded briefly in Chapter 3 to recent scholarly efforts to examine the negative impact of disease on national and international security; that is clearly an area of research that would benefit from further exploration—particularly systematic scientific analyses of a universal scope. However, much remains to be studied regarding the role of war as a determinant of population well-being, and I consider this book a useful step toward understanding the war-health relationship rather than the final word on that relationship. Effective evaluation of the social consequences of conflict would require continuous improvements in data on relevant public health, political, and economic factors, as well as deeper explorations of the multiple linkages between war and health. In addition to the elements of social decline discussed above, studies of post-conflict reconstruction would provide valuable insights into the manner in which conflict impacts the health of societies. The ability of a society to recover from conflict may have a significant influence on the degree to which its population health is affected, particularly in the long term. For example, the Iraqi society experienced continued deterioration in health achievement during the decade after the 1991 Gulf War due to its inability to rebuild important societal elements. Recovery from conflict includes establishment of viable political institutions, rebuilding of all aspects of infrastructure, and operation of social services such as health care and education at prewar levels.

As in all aspects of human security, the role of non-state actors holds prodigious importance in the war-health relationship. Involvement of international governmental and nongovernmental organizations is an important intervening factor in the social impact of war. A number of non-state actors also play a significant role in post-conflict reconstruction, influencing the ability of a state to achieve prewar levels of health. Therefore, another valuable direction for future research on this subject would be to examine the influence of international governmental and nongovernmental organizations on the conflict-health relationship. The difficulty in clearly explicating the relationship between war and health arises from the complexities of the relevant linkages, the challenge of identifying influential intervening factors, and the number of actors involved in ensuring the well-being of societies. Yet another direction to be explored in the relationship between armed conflict and health levels is the relative effects of war on the well-being of particular groups within societies. It is not unlikely for underprivileged groups within specific populations to be disproportionately affected by involvement in violent conflict, and it is a challenge to evaluate such differences in the consequences of conflict relying solely on country-level indicators. It is, therefore, necessary to continue examining the social and health consequences of violent conflict.

REFERENCE MATTER

APPENDIX A

The *World Health Report 2002*: Statistical Annex
Explanatory Notes

Annex Table 4 reports the average level of population health for WHO Member States in terms of healthy life expectancy. Based on more than 15 years of work, WHO introduced disability-adjusted life expectancy (DALE) as a summary measure of the level of health attained by populations in the *World Health Report 2000*. To better reflect the inclusion of all states of health in the calculation of healthy life expectancy, the name of the indicator used to measure healthy life expectancy has been changed from disability-adjusted life expectancy (DALE) to health-adjusted life expectancy (HALE). HALE is based on life expectancy at birth but includes an adjustment for time spent in poor health. It is most easily understood as the equivalent number of years in full health that a newborn can expect to live based on current rates of ill-health and mortality.

The measurement of time spent in poor health is based on combining condition-specific estimates from the Global Burden of Disease 2000 study with estimates of the prevalence of different health states by age and sex derived from health surveys. As noted above, for this year's *World Health Report*, burden of disease estimates of prevalences for specific diseases, injuries and their sequelae have been updated for many of the cause categories included in the Global Burden of Disease (GBD) 2000 study.

Analyses of over 50 national health surveys for the calculation of healthy life expectancy in the *World Health Report 2000* identified severe limitations in the comparability of self-reported health status data from different populations, even when identical survey instruments and methods are used. The WHO Household

Survey Study carried out 69 representative household surveys in 60 Member States in 2000 and 2001 using a new health status instrument based on the International Classification of Functioning, Disability and Health, which seeks information from a representative sample of respondents on their current states of health according to six core domains. These domains were identified from an extensive review of the currently available health status measurement instruments. To overcome the problem of comparability of self-report health data, the WHO survey instrument used performance tests and vignettes to calibrate self-reported health on selected domains such as cognition, mobility and vision. WHO has developed several statistical methods for correcting biases in self-reported health using these data, based on the hierarchical ordered probit (HOPIT) model. The calibrated responses are used to estimate the true prevalence of different states of health by age and sex.

Annex Table 4 reports average HALE at birth for Member States for 2000 and 2001, and for 2001 the following additional information: HALE at age 60, expected lost healthy years (LHE) at birth, per cent of total life expectancy lost, and 95 percent uncertainty intervals. LHE is calculated as life expectancy (LE) minus HALE and is the expected equivalent number of years of full health lost through living in health states of less than full health. The percentage of total life expectancy lost is LHE expressed as a percentage of total LE and represents the proportion of total life expectancy that is lost through living in health states of less than full health. HALEs for 2000 differ from those published in the *World Health Report 2001* for many Member States, as they incorporate new epidemiological information, new data from health surveys, and new information on mortality rates, as well as improvements in survey analysis methods.

The uncertainty ranges for healthy life expectancy given in Annex Table 4 are based on the 2.5th percentile and 97.5th percentile of the relevant uncertainty distributions. The ranges thus define 95 percent uncertainty intervals around the estimates. HALE uncertainty is a function of the uncertainty in age-specific mortality measurement for each country, of the uncertainty in burden of disease based estimates of country-level disability prevalence, and of uncertainty in the health state prevalences derived from health surveys.

Source: *World Health Report 2002*. Geneva: World Health Organization.

APPENDIX B

Calculation of Disability-Free Life Expectancy

	Ordinary Life Table			Disability Prevalence (%) $prev_X$	Years with Disability YD_X	Years Without Disability YWD_X	LE with Disability DLE_X	Disability-Free LE $DFLE_X$
Age	Survivors l_X	Years Lived L_X	Expectation of Life e_X					
0	100000	496210	74.98	4.5	22130	474080	16.60	58.38
5	99134	495425	70.63	9.6	47506	447919	16.52	54.11
10	99045	495018	65.69	8.6	42568	452450	16.05	49.64
15	98940	493916	60.76	5.7	28100	465816	15.64	45.12
20	98572	491448	55.98	7.6	37433	454015	15.41	40.56
25	97997	488469	51.29	8.5	41623	446846	15.12	36.17
30	97383	485285	46.60	10.6	51280	434005	14.79	31.81
35	96722	481816	41.90	12.2	59013	422803	14.36	27.54
40	95988	477781	37.20	14.3	68247	409534	13.86	23.34
45	95079	472220	32.53	17.9	84507	387713	13.27	19.26
50	93701	463324	27.97	23.5	108766	354558	12.57	15.40
55	91452	448652	23.59	30.9	138780	309872	11.68	11.90
60	87702	424469	19.48	41.6	176738	247731	10.60	8.88
65	81656	386806	15.73	44.0	170265	216541	9.22	6.50
70	72512	332217	12.38	58.3	193526	138691	8.04	4.34
75	59796	259645	9.45	59.6	154714	104931	6.51	2.94
80	43550	173081	7.02	73.2	126672	46409	5.39	1.63
85	25802	132424	5.13	81.5	107916	24508	4.18	0.95

NOTES: First four columns are from a standard life table for a population.

l_X is the number of survivors at age X in the hypothetical life table cohort.

L_X is the number of years of life lived by the life table cohort between ages X and X + 5.

$prev_X$ is the prevalence of disability between ages X and X + 5 in the population.

Years lived without disability $YD_X = L_X * prev_X$.

Years lived without disability $YWD_X = L_X * (1 - prev_X)$.

DLE_X = Sum of years lived with disability for ages x and above, divided by l_X.

$DFLE_X$ = Sum of years lived without disability for ages x and above, divided by l_X.

SOURCE: Mathers et al. 2001b.

APPENDIX C

Health-Adjusted Life Expectancy (HALE), 1999–2002

Country	1999	2000	2001	2002
Afghanistan	37.7	33.8	33.4	35.5
Albania	60.0	58.6	58.7	61.4
Algeria	61.6	57.5	57.8	60.6
Andorra	72.3	70.8	70.9	72.2
Angola	38.0	28.9	28.7	33.4
Antigua and Barbuda	65.8	59.7	59.7	61.9
Argentina	66.7	62.9	63.1	65.3
Armenia	66.7	57.9	58.3	61.0
Australia	73.2	71.4	71.6	72.6
Austria	71.6	70.7	71.0	71.4
Azerbaijan	63.7	51.7	52.8	57.2
Bahamas	59.1	58.4	58.6	63.5
Bahrain	64.4	61.9	61.8	64.3
Bangladesh	49.9	52.0	52.1	54.3
Barbados	65.0	63.9	64.3	65.6
Belarus	61.7	58.8	58.4	60.7
Belgium	71.6	69.6	69.7	71.1
Belize	60.9	58.7	58.9	60.3
Benin	42.2	42.1	42.1	44.0
Bhutan	51.8	51.2	51.4	52.9
Bolivia	53.3	50.4	50.8	54.4
Bosnia and Herzegovina	64.9	62.3	62.5	64.3
Botswana	32.3	34.4	32.9	35.7
Brazil	59.1	56.3	56.7	59.8
Brunei Darussalam	64.4	62.0	62.0	65.3
Bulgaria	64.4	63.1	63.0	64.8

(continued)

Appendix C. (continued)

Country	1999	2000	2001	2002
Burkina Faso	35.5	35.0	35.1	35.6
Burundi	34.6	33.9	33.7	35.1
Cambodia	45.7	45.9	46.4	47.5
Cameroon	42.2	41.0	40.4	41.5
Canada	72.0	69.7	69.9	72.0
Cape Verde	57.6	56.3	56.5	60.8
Central African Republic	36.0	34.0	34.0	37.4
Chad	39.4	38.5	38.7	40.7
Chile	68.6	65.8	66.1	67.3
China	62.3	62.8	63.2	64.1
Colombia	62.9	58.6	58.7	62.0
Comoros	46.8	49.7	49.9	54.6
Congo	45.1	42.9	43.0	46.3
Cook Islands		60.4	60.5	61.6
Costa Rica	66.7	65.0	64.8	67.2
Cote d'Ivoire	42.8	38.0	37.8	39.5
Croatia	67.0	63.1	63.3	66.6
Cuba	68.4	66.6	66.6	68.3
Cyprus	69.8	66.2	66.2	67.6
Czech Republic	68.0	66.4	66.6	68.4
Democratic People's Republic of Korea	52.3	55.8	55.8	58.8
Democratic Republic of the Congo	36.3	34.9	34.8	37.1
Denmark	69.4	69.8	70.1	69.8
Djibouti	37.9	39.9	40.1	42.9
Dominica	69.8	62.0	62.1	63.7
Dominican Republic	62.5	56.0	56.4	59.6
Ecuador	61.0	59.0	59.5	61.9
Egypt	58.5	56.4	56.7	59.0
El Salvador	61.5	56.8	57.4	59.7
Equatorial Guinea	44.1	43.6	43.8	45.5
Eritrea	33.5	37.5	44.1	50.0
Estonia	59.4	61.9	62.0	64.1
Ethiopia	70.5	38.5	38.8	41.2
Fiji	59.4	58.7	58.8	58.8
Finland	70.5	69.9	70.1	71.1
France	73.1	71.1	71.3	72.0
Gabon	47.8	49.7	49.9	51.4
Gambia	48.3	47.8	48.0	49.5
Georgia	66.3	59.7	59.8	64.4
Germany	70.4	70.1	70.2	71.8
Ghana	45.5	47.7	47.8	49.8
Greece	72.5	70.4	70.4	71.0
Grenada	65.5	57.3	57.5	59.2
Guatemala	54.3	54.0	54.3	57.4
Guinea	37.8	42.0	42.4	44.8
Guinea-Bissau	37.2	38.3	38.3	40.5
Guyana	60.2	53.5	54.1	55.2
Haiti	43.8	45.1	42.9	43.8
Honduras	61.1	55.7	55.9	58.4

(continued)

Appendix C. (continued)

Country	1999	2000	2001	2002
Hungary	64.1	64.1	61.8	64.9
Iceland	70.8	70.8	71.2	72.8
India	60.5	53.2	51.4	53.5
Indonesia	55.3	59.7	56.7	58.1
Iran, Islamic Republic of	69.6	60.5	56.7	57.6
Iraq	70.4	55.3	50.5	50.1
Ireland	72.7	69.6	69.0	69.8
Israel	67.3	70.4	69.4	71.4
Italy	74.5	72.7	71.0	72.7
Jamaica	60.0	67.3	62.8	65.1
Japan	74.5	73.5	73.6	75.0
Jordan	60.0	58.5	58.5	61.0
Kazakhstan	56.4	52.1	52.4	55.9
Kenya	39.3	41.4	40.8	44.4
Kiribati		52.9	53.2	54.0
Kuwait	63.2	65.1	64.9	67.1
Kyrgyzstan	56.3	51.4	51.5	55.3
Lao People's Democratic Republic	46.1	44.2	44.2	47.0
Latvia	62.2	59.9	60.0	62.8
Lebanon	60.6	59.2	59.4	60.4
Lesotho	36.9	34.9	33.4	31.4
Liberia	34.0	37.0	37.5	35.3
Libyan Arab Jamahiriya	59.3	59.3	59.6	63.7
Lithuania	64.1	60.8	61.1	63.3
Luxembourg	71.1	70.3	70.6	71.5
Madagascar	36.6	44.4	44.5	48.6
Malawi	29.4	30.1	29.8	34.9
Malaysia	61.4	60.5	60.4	63.2
Maldives	53.9	51.1	51.9	57.8
Mali	33.1	35.6	35.7	37.9
Malta	70.5	69.2	69.2	71.4
Marshall Islands		52.3	52.6	54.8
Mauritania	41.4	41.5	41.6	44.5
Mauritius	62.7	57.2	57.1	62.4
Mexico	65.0	63.8	63.8	65.4
Micronesia, Federated States of		55.5	55.8	57.7
Monaco	72.4	70.8	71.3	72.9
Mongolia	53.8	53.7	53.9	55.6
Morocco	59.1	55.3	55.4	60.2
Mozambique	34.4	36.3	36.0	36.9
Myanmar	51.6	48.9	48.9	51.7
Namibia	35.6	41.8	40.4	43.3
Nauru		52.5	52.7	55.1
Nepal	49.5	48.7	48.9	51.8
Netherlands	72.0	69.7	69.9	71.2
New Zealand	69.2	70.1	70.3	70.8
Nicaragua	58.1	57.7	57.8	61.4

(continued)

Appendix C. (continued)

Country	1999	2000	2001	2002
Niger	29.1	33.1	33.2	35.5
Nigeria	38.3	41.9	41.9	41.5
Niue		59.2	59.1	60.4
Norway	71.7	70.7	70.8	72.0
Oman	63.0	60.4	60.4	64.0
Pakistan	55.9	50.9	50.9	53.3
Palau	59.0	57.4	57.7	59.6
Panama	66.0	63.9	64.1	66.2
Papua New Guinea	47.0	49.6	49.8	51.9
Paraguay	63.0	58.4	58.7	61.9
Peru	59.4	57.1	57.4	61.0
Philippines	58.9	55.2	55.5	59.3
Poland	66.2	64.3	64.3	65.8
Portugal	69.3	66.8	66.8	69.2
Qatar	63.5	61.2	61.2	65.2
Republic of Korea	65.0	67.2	67.4	67.8
Republic of Moldova	61.5	57.3	57.5	59.8
Romania	62.3	61.0	60.9	63.1
Russian Federation	61.3	56.6	56.7	58.4
Rwanda	32.8	34.1	33.8	38.3
Saint Kitts and Nevis	61.6	60.7	60.8	61.5
Saint Lucia	65.0	60.4	60.6	62.7
Saint Vincent and the Grenadines	66.4	59.8	59.8	61.0
Samoa		57.8	57.7	59.7
San Marino	72.3	72.1	72.2	73.4
São Tomé and Principe	53.5	51.2	51.4	54.4
Saudi Arabia	64.5	59.8	60.0	61.4
Senegal	44.6	45.3	45.4	48.0
Seychelles	59.3	59.0	59.1	61.2
Sierra Leone	25.9	25.8	26.5	28.6
Singapore	69.3	68.5	68.7	70.1
Slovakia	66.6	64.1	64.1	66.2
Slovenia	68.4	67.5	67.7	69.5
Solomon Islands	54.9	54.6	54.8	56.2
Somalia	36.4	35.1	35.0	36.8
South Africa	39.8	43.0	41.3	44.3
Spain	72.8	70.7	70.9	72.6
Sri Lanka	62.8	58.3	58.9	61.6
Sudan	43.0	45.9	45.5	48.5
Suriname	62.7	57.2	57.5	58.8
Swaziland	38.1	35.4	33.9	34.2
Sweden	73.0	71.6	71.8	73.3
Switzerland	72.5	72.5	72.8	73.2
Syria	58.8	59.0	59.2	61.7
Tajikistan	57.3	49.4	50.1	54.7
Thailand	60.2	58.6	58.6	60.1
The former Yugoslav Republic of Macedonia	63.7	62.3	62.2	63.4
Togo	40.7	42.8	42.7	44.6
Tonga		59.0	58.8	61.8

(continued)

Appendix C. (continued)

Country	1999	2000	2001	2002
Trinidad and Tobago	64.6	60.4	60.4	62.0
Tunisia	61.4	61.1	61.3	62.5
Turkey	62.9	59.7	59.8	62.0
Turkmenistan	54.3	50.2	50.3	54.4
Tuvalu		53.9	53.9	53.0
Uganda	32.7	37.5	38.0	42.7
Ukraine	63.0	57.5	57.4	59.2
United Arab Emirates	65.4	62.4	62.5	63.9
United Kingdom	71.7	69.2	69.6	70.6
United Republic of Tanzania	36.0	37.8	37.8	40.4
United States	70.0	67.4	67.6	69.3
Uruguay	67.0	64.7	64.7	66.2
Uzbekistan	60.2	53.4	53.5	59.4
Vanuatu	52.8	54.6	54.9	58.9
Venezuela, Bolivarian Republic of	65.0	60.9	61.1	64.2
Viet Nam	58.2	58.5	58.6	61.3
Yemen	49.7	47.9	48.4	49.3
Yugoslavia	66.1	62.0	62.1	
Zambia	30.3	31.1	30.9	34.9
Zimbabwe	32.9	32.0	31.3	33.6

SOURCE: World Health Organization, "Global Burden of Disease Project."

NOTES

1. For a detailed discussion of the goals and purposes of human security, see the Commission on Human Security (2003). This report presents human security as the appropriate paradigm for understanding global security and adheres to a broad and holistic conceptualization of human security.

2. See Austin and Bruch (2000) for multidisciplinary perspectives on the environmental consequences of violent conflict, including legal, ecological, and public health effects.

3. A previous version of the theoretical arguments and empirical analyses presented in this chapter was published as Zaryab Iqbal, "Health and Human Security: The Public Health Impact of Violent Conflict," *International Studies Quarterly* 50(3) (2006): 631–649.

4. Appendix A contains a longer excerpt from the WHO *World Health Report 2002* that explains the logic of the HALE measure as well as the data-collection and computation methods involved in deriving this measure.

5. The *Education* variable is not included in the second model, which assesses the relationship between short-term changes in the covariates and HALE, because the education measure used here does not change on a yearly basis.

6. A possible influence on health achievement that has not been included in these models is a state's health care capacity. States with larger health care capacities—including hospitals, health care personnel, and medical supplies—are likely to have higher HALEs. However, health care infrastructure—as well as general infrastructure—can be damaged or even destroyed due to violent conflict (Ghobarah et al. 2004). In fact, it is not uncommon for health care facilities to be targeted during combat. As a result, controlling for this variable in the models in Tables 4.3 and 4.4 would confound the influence of the primary covariate of interest, conflict.

Ray (2003) warns against controlling for intervening variables or including independent variables that are related to each other. I did, however, estimate alternative models using immunization rates as a proxy for health care capacity, but this variable did not have any significant effect.

7. Approximately 25 percent of the states for which HALE is available were not included in the analysis due to missing data, mainly on economic variables. The states that were excluded from the analysis experienced significantly higher levels of intense conflict than the countries that were included in the model, and bivariate analyses reveal that the negative relationship between conflict and health is considerably stronger in the group of states excluded from the analysis than in the included group. Thus, the exclusion of states with high levels of conflict likely mitigated the effect of conflict on HALE as revealed by the results in Table 4.3, and the negative relationship between conflict and health would be stronger if those states were included in the analysis.

8. It should be noted, as in Ghobarah et al. (2004), that some of the states with observed health outcome levels that are significantly lower than their expected HALE have high HIV prevalence rates. These outliers include South Africa, Namibia, Botswana, Swaziland, Zimbabwe, and Zambia. High levels of HIV/AIDS prevalence could have clear repercussions for health achievement. Moreover, arguments have been made about the contribution of conditions created by civil wars in sub-Saharan Africa to an increase in HIV/AIDS rates.

9. Both this model and the model assessing short-term changes in health were also estimated using a dichotomized measure of democracy, in which states with a POLITY IV score of 5 or higher were considered democracies and those with a score lower than 5 were considered nondemocracies. The results with this dichotomous measure of democracy were very similar in significance to the models shown, with a higher coefficient and a higher standard error.

10. As explained in Chapter 4, the POLITY scores range from −10 to 10, with higher scores denoting higher levels of democracy. A state with a score of 10 is at the highest level of democracy and one with a score of −10 is an autocracy.

11. Data on GDP and trade come from the Penn World Table (Heston et al. 2002).

12. The *Population* variable reflects the population of states in millions in a given year. Population figures come from the World Development Indicators (World Bank 2004).

13. The countries of Oceania—including Australia and New Zealand—have been included in Europe and North America for this analysis due to similar political, cultural, and economic characteristics.

14. Cahill (1999) presents a number of essays on the influence of international humanitarian assistance on conflict-ridden societies, with particular attention to the mitigating effect of such intervention on the health consequences of conflict and other disasters.

15. Note that, throughout this analysis, I treat war as strongly exogenous. For a contrary position that asserts that war can be a consequence of health, see, *inter alia*, Peterson and Shellman 2006 and Price-Smith 2001, 2009.

16. For the analysis in Table 7.1, I use economic data from the Penn World Tables (Heston et al. 2002); these data include per-capita GDP for each state in constant dollars and the government share of the GDP. To assess the presence of conflict, I consult data from the Peace Research Institute of Oslo (PRIO) on armed conflict (Gleditsch et al. 2002). These data measure conflict according to both its intensity and its type, including domestic and international conflict. I categorize conflict as major and minor conflict. Major conflict refers to militarized conflicts that result in at least 1,000 battle deaths in a given year; minor conflicts refers to conflicts in which there have been at least 25 deaths in a given year and more than 1,000 deaths in the history of the conflict (the PRIO dataset refers to these conflicts as *intermediate*).

17. In this analysis minor conflict corresponds to the definition for intermediate conflict in the PRIO dataset.

18. Although a large proportion of forced migrants are internally displaced persons (IDPs) as a result of armed conflict, this analysis focuses on the effects of refugee flows on the health outcomes in the host state. For a discussion of the global issue of internal displacement, see Cohen and Deng 1998.

19. The large-scale refugee flows from Afghanistan to Pakistan following the Soviet invasion in 1979 was an exception to the trend in refugee flows identified here. As of 2005, there were still 2 million Afghans living in Pakistan and Iran (United Nations High Commissioner for Refugees 2005).

20. Weiner (1992) discusses the destabilizing effects of mass migration in general and does not focus entirely on refugee flows. However, his arguments do indeed apply to forced migration, and he includes a specific discussion of the effects of refugee flows, particularly with respect to the relationship between the refugees' home and host states.

21. For an analysis of mortality among large refugee groups, including methods for mortality surveillance in complex emergencies, see National Research Council (2001), *Forced Migration and Mortality*.

22. In an analysis of mortality among Rwandan refugees in various parts of Zaire, Legros et al. (2001) state that in July 1994, following an influx of refugees

into the Katale, Kibumba, and Mugunga camps, 58,000 to 80,000 cases of cholera were reported within a month and roughly 50,000 deaths occurred during that one-month period.

23. Only states that received at least one refugee were included in the sample used for this scatter plot.

24. For a more detailed explanation of this refugee measure, see the online appendix to Moore and Shellman (2007). For discussion of quality issues in forced migration data, see Crisp (2000) and Schmeidl (2000).

25. As in other analyses in the book, the conflict data were obtained from the Peace Research Institute of Oslo (PRIO) data set on armed conflict (Gleditsch et al. 2002), and the same operationalization of the variables is employed as in previous chapters.

26. A state's democracy level is measured by its POLITY IV score (Marshall and Jaggers 2004), which ranges from -10 to 10. The data for the economic variables, *Per-Capita GDP* and *Trade Openness*, and *Population* were acquired from the Penn World Table (Heston et al. 2002).

27. The first-stage equation of the instrumental variables models, while not presented here, are available upon request from the author. Because all first-stage models have identical model specifications and differ only in the number of observation used in their estimation, all yield substantively similar findings; accordingly, I summarize them briefly here. The models exhibit a moderately strong fit, with an R^2 around 0.3. The instrumental variable of refugee flows at a two-year lag shows a very large and statistically significant impact on refugee flows at a one-year lag. Also, as expected, major conflict is associated with higher levels of refugee flows, although there is no significant effect of minor conflict. Per-capita GDP, population, and year lead to an increase in refugee flows; these findings are consistent with arguments in previous work regarding the propensity of refugees to migrate to states with higher income levels and larger populations (e.g., Iqbal 2007). Democracy and economic openness in a host state do not seem to influence refugee flows.

REFERENCES

Achen, Christopher. 2000. "Why Lagged Dependent Variables Can Suppress the Explanatory Power of Other Independent Variables." Paper presented at the Annual Meeting of the Political Methodology Section of the American Political Science Association, UCLA, July 20–22.

Aitchison, John. 1986. *The Statistical Analysis of Compositional Data.* London: Chapman and Hall.

Alkire, Sabina. 2002. "Conceptual Framework for the Commission on Human Security." Available at www.humansecurity-chs.org/doc/frame.html.

Alston, Philip, ed. 1992. *The United Nations and Human Rights: A Critical Appraisal.* Oxford: Oxford University Press.

Annan, Kofi. 2000. "Secretary-General Salutes International Workshop on Human Security in Mongolia," two-day session in Ulaanbaatar, May 8–10. Press Release SG/SM/7382.

Apostolakis, Bobby E. 1992. "Warfare-Welfare Expenditure Substitution in Latin America, 1953–87." *Journal of Peace Research* 29(1): 85–98.

Austin, Jay E. and Carl E. Bruch, eds. 2000. *The Environmental Consequences of War: Legal, Economic, and Scientific Perspectives.* Cambridge: Cambridge University Press.

Bacci, Massimo Livi. 2001. "Comment: Desired Family Size and the Future Course of Fertility." *Population and Development Review* 27(Supplement: Global Fertility Transition): 282–289.

Baum, Matthew and David A. Lake. 2003. "The Political Economy of Growth: Democracy and Human Capital." *American Journal of Political Science* 47(20): 333–347.

Bigombe, Betty, Paul Collier, and Nicholas Sambanis. 2000. "Policies for Building Post-Conflict Peace." *Journal of African Economies* 9(3): 322–347.

Boutros-Ghali, Boutros. 1992. *An Agenda for Peace: Preventive Diplomacy, Peacemaking and Peacekeeping: Report of the Secretary-General.* UN GAOR/ SCOR, 47th Session, Preliminary List Item 10, at 55, UN Docs. A/47/277 and S/2411.

Bruderlein, Claude. 2001. "People's Security as a New Measure of Global Security." *International Review of the Red Cross* 842(June): 353–366.

Brundtland, Gro Harlem. 2003. "The Globalization of Health." *Seton Hall Journal of Diplomacy and International Relations* 4(2): 7–12.

Bueno de Mesquita, Bruce and Randolph M. Siverson. 1995. "War and the Survival of Political Leaders: A Comparative Study of Regime Types and Political Accountability." *American Political Science Review* 89(4): 841–855.

Bueno de Mesquita, Bruce and Randolph M. Siverson. 1997. "Nasty or Nice? Political Systems, Endogenous Norms, and the Treatment of Adversaries." *Journal of Conflict Resolution* (New Games: Modeling Domestic-International Linkages) 41(1): 175–199.

Bueno de Mesquita, Bruce, Randolph Siverson, and Gary Wollers. 1992. "War and the Fate of Regimes: A Comparative Analysis." *American Political Science Review* 86(3): 638–646.

Bueno de Mesquita, Bruce, Alastair Smith, Randolph M. Siverson, and James D. Morrow. 2003. *The Logic of Political Survival.* Cambridge, MA: MIT Press.

Cahill, Kevin M., ed. 1999. *A Framework for Survival: Health, Human Rights, and Humanitarian Assistance in Conflicts and Disasters.* London: Routledge.

Caldwell, John. 1979. "Education as a Factor in Mortality Decline: An Examination of Nigerian Data." *Population Studies* 33(3): 395–413.

Caldwell, John. 2001. "The Globalization of Fertility Behavior." *Population and Development Review* 27(Supplement: Global Fertility Transition): 93–115.

Carballo, Manuel and Aditi Nerukar. 2001. "Migration, Refugees, and Health Risks." *Emerging Infectious Diseases* 7(3: Supplement): 556–560.

Cleland, John. 2001. "The Effects of Improved Survival of Fertility: A Reassessment." *Population and Development Review* 27(Supplement: Global Fertility Transition): 60–92.

Cohen, Roberta and Francis M. Deng. 1998. *Masses in Flight: The Global Crisis of Internal Displacement.* Washington, DC: The Brookings Institute.

Collier, Paul. 1999. "On the Economic Consequences of Civil War." *Oxford Economic Papers* 51: 168–183.

Commission on Human Security. 2003. *Human Security Now.* New York: Commission on Human Security.

Crisp, Jeff. 2000. "Who Has Counted the Refugees? UNHCR and the Politics of Numbers." In Stephen C. Lubkemann, Larry Minear, and Thomas G. Weiss, eds., *Humanitarian Action: Social Science Connections.* Providence, RI: Thomas J. Watson Jr. Institute for International Studies, 33–62.

Davenport, Christian A., Will H. Moore, and Steven C. Poe. 2003. "Sometimes You Just Have to Leave: Domestic Threats and Forced Migration, 1964–1989." *International Interactions* 29: 27–55.

Davis, David R. and Steve Chan. 1990. "The Security Welfare Relationship: Longitudinal Evidence from Taiwan." *Journal of Peace Research* 27: 87–100.

Davis, David R. and Joel N. Kuritsky. 2002. "Violent Conflict and Its Impact on Health Indicators in Sub-Saharan Africa, 1980 to 1997." Paper presented at the Annual Meeting of the International Studies Association, New Orleans, LA, March.

Dickie, Mark and Shelby Gerking. 2000. "Valuing Public Health Damages Arising from War." In Jay E. Austin and Carl E. Bruch, eds., *The Environmental Consequences of War: Legal, Economic, and Scientific Perspectives.* Cambridge: Cambridge University Press, 501–529.

Domke, William K., Richard C. Eichenberg, and Catherine M. Kelleher. 1983. "The Illusion of Choice: Defense and Welfare in Advanced Industrial Democracies, 1948–1978." *American Political Science Review* 77(1): 19–35.

Elbe, Stefan. 2002. "HIV/AIDS and the Changing Landscape of War in Africa." *International Security* 27(2): 159–177.

Elbe, Stefan. 2003. "Health, Strategy and HIV/AIDS." In Stefan Elbe, ed., *Strategic Implications of HIV/AIDS.* New York: Oxford University Press, 13–21.

Evans, David B., Ajay Tandon, Christopher Murray, and Jeremy Lauer. 2001. "Comparative Efficiency of National Health Systems: Cross National Econometric Analysis." *British Medical Journal* 323(7308): 307–310.

Fargues, Philippe. 2000. "Protracted National Conflict and Fertility Change: Palestinians and Israelis in the Twentieth Century." *Population and Development Review* 26(3): 441–482.

Fitzgerald, Valpy. 2001. "Paying for the War: Economic Policy in Poor Countries Under Conflict Conditions." In Frances Stewart and Valpy Fitzgerald, eds., *War and Underdevelopment,* vol. 1: *The Economic and Social Consequences of Conflict.* New York: Oxford University Press, 21–38.

Flegg, A. T. 1982. "Inequality of Income, Illiteracy and Medical Care as Determinants of Infant Mortality in Underdeveloped Countries." *Population Studies* 36(3): 441–458.

Foege, William H. 1997. "Arms and Public Health: A Global Perspective." In Barry S. Levy and Victor W. Sidel, eds., *War and Public Health.* New York: Oxford University Press, 3–11.

Garfield, Richard and Alfred I. Neugut. 1997. "The Human Consequences of War." In Barry S. Levy and Victor W. Sidel, eds., *War and Public Health*. New York: Oxford University Press, 27–38.

Ghobarah, Hazem, Paul Huth, and Bruce Russett. 2003. "Civil Wars Kill and Maim People Long After the Shooting Stops." *American Political Science Review* 97(2): 189–202.

Ghobarah, Hazem, Paul Huth, Bruce Russett, and Gary King. 2004. "The Political Economy of Comparative Human Misery and Well-Being." *International Studies Quarterly* 48(1): 73–94.

Gilpin, Robert. 1981. *War and Change in World Politics*. London: Cambridge University Press.

Gleditsch, Nils Petter, Peter Wallensteen, Mikael Eriksson, Margareta Sollenberg, and Havard Strand. 2002. "Armed Conflict 1946–2001: A New Dataset." *Journal of Peace Research* 39(5): 615–637.

Goemans, Hein. 2000a. "Fighting for Survival: The Fate of Leaders and the Duration of War." *Journal of Conflict Resolution* 44(5): 555–579.

Goemans, Hein. 2000b. *War and Punishment: The Causes of War Termination and the First World War*. Princeton, NJ: Princeton University Press.

Goulding, Marrack. 1993. "The Evolution of United Nations Peacekeeping." *International Affairs* 69(3): 451–464.

Gruskin, Sofia and Daniel Tarantola. 2005. "Health and Human Rights." In Sophia Gruskin, Michael A. Grodin, George J. Annas, and Stephen P. Parks, eds., *Perspectives on Health and Human Rights*. New York: Routledge Taylor and Francis Group, 3–58.

Gyimah-Brempong, Kwabena. 1992. "Do African Governments Favor Defense in Budgeting?" *Journal of Peace Research* 29(2): 191–206.

Hampson, Fen Osler and John B. Hay. 2003. "Human Security: A Review of the Scholarly Literature." Working paper.

Heston, Alan, Robert Summers, and Bettina Aten. 2002. *Penn World Table Version 6.1*. Philadelphia: Center for International Comparisons of Production, Income and Prices at the University of Pennsylvania (CICUP).

Heston, Alan, Robert Summers, and Bettina Aten. 2006. *Penn World Table Version 6.2*. Philadelphia: Center for International Comparisons of Production, Income and Prices at the University of Pennsylvania.

Hoskins, Eric. 1997. "Public Health and the Persian Gulf War." In Barry S. Levy and Victor W. Sidel, eds., *War and Public Health*. New York: Oxford University Press, 254–280.

International Monetary Fund. 1993. *Government Financial Statistics Yearbook*. Washington, DC: International Monetary Fund.

Iqbal, Zaryab. 2006. "Health and Human Security: The Public Health Impact of Violent Conflict." *International Studies Quarterly* 50(3): 631–649.

Iqbal, Zaryab. 2007. "The Geo-Politics of Forced Migration in Africa, 1992–2001." *Conflict Resolution and Peace Science* 24: 105–119.

Iqbal, Zaryab and Christopher Zorn. 2007. "Civil War and Refugees in Post–Cold War Africa." *Civil Wars* 9(2): 200–213.

Iqbal, Zaryab and Christopher Zorn. 2010. "Violent Conflict and the Spread of HIV/AIDS in Africa." *Journal of Politics* (forthcoming).

Katz, Jonathan N. and Gary King. 1999. "A Statistical Model for Multiparty Electoral Data." *American Political Science Review* 93(1): 15–32.

Kawachi, Ichiro, Bruce P. Kennedy, Kimberly Lochner, and Deborah Prothrow-Stith. 1997. "Social Capital, Income Inequality, and Mortality." *American Journal of Public Health* 87(9): 1491–1498.

King, Gary and Lisa L. Martin. 2001. "The Human Costs of Military Conflict." Overview paper presented at the Conference on Military Conflict as a Public Health Problem, Cambridge, MA, September 29.

King, Gary and Christopher J. L. Murray. 2002. "Rethinking Human Security." *Political Science Quarterly* 116(4): 585–610.

Krause, Keith and Michael C. Williams. 1996. "Broadening the Agenda of Security Studies: Politics and Methods." *Mershon International Studies Review* 40(2): 229–254.

Lauren, Paul Gordon. 1998. *The Evolution of Human International Rights: Visions Seen.* University Park: Pennsylvania State University Press.

Leaning, Jennifer, Susan M. Briggs, and Lincoln C. Chen, eds. 1999. *Humanitarian Crises: The Medical and Public Health Response.* Cambridge, MA: Harvard University Press.

Legros, Dominique, Christophe Paquet, and Pierre Nabeth. 2001. "The Evolution of Mortality Among Rwanda Refugees in Zaire Between 1994 and 1997." In National Research Council, *Forced Migration and Mortality.* Roundtable of the Demography of Forced Migration, Committee on Population, Holly E. Reed and Charles B. Keely, eds. Commission on Behavioral and Social Sciences and Education. Washington, DC: National Academy Press, 52–68.

Leon, David A. and Gill Walt, eds. 2001. *Poverty, Inequality, and Health: An International Perspective.* New York: Oxford University Press.

Levy, Barry S. and Victor W. Sidel, eds. 1997. *War and Public Health.* New York: Oxford University Press.

Levy, Barry S. and Victor W. Sidel. 2002. "The Health and Social Consequences of Diversion of Economic Resources to War and Preparation for War." In Ilkka Taipale, ed., *War or Health? A Reader.* London: Zed Books, 208–221.

Liang, Kung-Yee and Scott L. Zeger. 1986. "Longitudinal Data Analysis Using Generalized Linear Models." *Biometrika* 73(1): 13–22.

Lodgaard, Sverre. 2000. "Human Security: Concept and Operationalization." Paper prepared for "Expert Seminar on Human Rights and Peace," Geneva, December 8–9.

Mack, Andrew. 2001. "Notes on the Creation of a Human Security Report." Paper presented at a conference at the Kennedy School of Government, Harvard University, December 1–2.

Marshall, Monty G. and Keith Jaggers. 2004. *POLITY IV Project.* Integrated Network for Societal Conflict Research Program and Center for International Development and Conflict Management, University of Maryland, College Park.

Marshall, Monty G. and Keith Jaggers. 2009. *POLITY IV Project: Political Regime Characteristics and Transitions, 1800–2007.* Center for Global Policy, School of Public Policy, George Mason University, Fairfax, VA, and Center for Systemic Peace, Severn, MD.

Mathers, Colin D., Ritu Sadana, Joshua A. Salomon, Christopher J. L. Murray, and Alan D. Lopez. 2000. "Estimates of DALE for 191 Countries: Methods and Results." *Global Programme on Evidence for Health Policy*, World Health Organization, Working Paper No. 16.

Mathers, Colin D., Ritu Sadana, Joshua A. Salomon, Christopher J. L. Murray, and Alan D. Lopez. 2001a. "Healthy Life Expectancy in 191 Countries, 1999." *Lancet* 357: 1685–1691.

Mathers, Colin D., T. Vos, Alan D. Lopez, Joshua Salomon, and M. Ezzati, eds. 2001b. *National Burden of Disease Studies: A Practical Guide.* Edition 2.0. Global Program on Evidence for Health Policy. Geneva: World Health Organization.

McPherson, James. 1988. *Battle Cry of Freedom: The Civil War Era.* New York: Oxford University Press.

McRae, Rob and Don Hubert, eds. 2002. *Human Security and the New Diplomacy: Protecting People, Promoting Peace.* Montreal: McGill–Queen's University Press.

Michaud, Catherine, Christopher Murray, and Barry Bloom. 2001. "Burden of Disease—Implications for Future Research." *Journal of American Medical Association* 285(5): 535–539.

Mintz, Alex. 1989. "Guns Versus Butter: A Disaggregated Analysis." *American Political Science Review* 83(4): 1285–1293.

Mintz, Alex and Chi Huang. 1990. "Defense Expenditures, Economic Growth, and the 'Peace Dividend.' " *American Political Science Review* 84(4): 1283–1293.

Mintz, Alex and Chi Huang. 1991. "Guns Versus Butter: The Indirect Link." *American Journal of Political Science* 35(3): 738–757.

Mintz, Alex and Michael D. Ward. 1989. "The Political Economy of Military Spending in Israel." *American Political Science Review* 83(2): 521–533.

Mitchell, Sara McLaughlin, Scott Gates, and Havard Hegre. 1999. "Evolution in Democracy-War Dynamics." *Journal of Conflict Resolution* 43(6): 771–792.

Moore, Jonathan. 1996. *The UN and Complex Emergencies: Rehabilitation in Third World Transitions.* Geneva: United Nations Research Institute for Social Development.

Moore, Will H. and Stephen M. Shellman. 2004. "Fear of Persecution: Forced Migration, 1952–1995." *Journal of Conflict Resolution* 40(5): 723–745.

Moore, Will H. and Stephen M. Shellman. 2007. "Whither Will They Go? A Global Study of Refugees' Destinations, 1965–1995." *International Studies Quarterly* 51: 811–834.

Morsink, Johannes. 1998. *The Universal Declaration of Human Rights: Origins, Drafting and Intent.* University Park: University of Pennsylvania Press.

Mousseau, Michael and Yuhang Shi. 1999. "A Test for Reverse Causality in the Democratic Peace Relationship." *Journal of Peace Research* 36(6): 639–663.

Murray, Christopher, Joshua A. Salomon, and Colin Mathers. 2000. "A Critical Examination of Summary Measures of Population Health." *Bulletin of the World Health Organization* 78(8): 981–994.

Murray, Christopher J. L., Gary King, Alan D. Lopez, N. Tomijima, and E. G. Krug. 2002. "Armed Conflict as a Public Health Problem." *British Medical Journal* 324 (February 9): 346–349.

National Research Council. 2001. *Forced Migration and Mortality.* Roundtable of the Demography of Forced Migration, Committee on Population, Holly E. Reed and Charles B. Keely, eds. Commission on Behavioral and Social Sciences and Education. Washington, DC: National Academy Press.

Noormahomed, Abdul Razak and Julie Cliff. 2002. "Health and War in Mozambique." In Ilkka Taipale, ed., *War or Health? A Reader.* London: Zed Books, 222–230.

Organski, A. F. K. and Jacek Kugler. 1980. *The War Ledger.* Chicago: University of Chicago Press.

Ostergard, Robert. 2002. "Politics in the Hot Zone: AIDS and the Threat to Africa's Security." *Third World Quarterly* 23(2): 333–350.

Paris, Roland. 2001. "Human Security: Paradigm Shift or Hot Air?" *International Security* 26(2): 87–102.

Pedersen, Duncan. 2002. "Political Violence, Ethnic Conflict, and Contemporary Wars: Broad Implications for Health and Social Well-Being." *Social Science and Medicine* 55: 175–190.

Peterson, Susan and Stephen Shellman. 2006. "AIDS and Violent Conflict: The Indirect Effects of Disease on National Security." Working paper, College of William and Mary.

Posen, Barry R. 1996. "Military Responses to Refugee Disasters." *International Security* 21(1): 72–111.

Price-Smith, Andrew T. 2001. *The Health of Nations: Infectious Disease, Environmental Change, and Their Effects on National Security and Development.* Cambridge, MA: MIT Press.

Price-Smith, Andrew T. 2003. "Praetoria's Shadow: The HIV/AIDS Pandemic and National Security in South Africa." Special Report 4, Health and Security Series. Washington, DC: Chemical and Biological Arms Control Institute.

Price-Smith, Andrew T. 2009. *Disease, Ecology, and National Security in the Era of Globalization.* Cambridge, MA: MIT Press.

Price-Smith, Andrew T. and John L. Daly. 2004. "Downward Spiral: HIV/AIDS, State Capacity, and Political Conflict in Zimbabwe." Peaceworks 53. Washington, DC: United States Institute of Peace.

Raheem, Kolawole T. and Kingsley K. Akinroye. 2002. "Warfare and Health: The Case of West Africa." In Ilkka Taipale, ed., *War or Health? A Reader.* London: Zed Books, 240–248.

Rasler, Karen and William R. Thompson. 1983. "Global Wars, Public Debts, and the Long Cycle." *World Politics* 35(4): 489–516.

Rasler, Karen and William R. Thompson. 1985. "War and the Economic Growth of Major Powers." *American Journal of Political Science* 29(3): 513–538.

Rasler, Karen and William R. Thompson. 1988. "Defense Burdens, Capital Formation, and Economic Growth: The Systemic Leader Case." *Journal of Conflict Resolution* 32(1): 61–86.

Ray, James Lee. 2003. "Explaining Interstate Conflict and War: What Should Be Controlled For?" *Conflict Management and Peace Science* 20(2): 1–23.

Reiter, Dan. 2001. "Does Peace Nurture Democracy?" *Journal of Politics* 63(3): 935–948.

Rodgers, G. B. 1979. "Income and Inequality as Determinants of Mortality: An International Cross-Section Analysis." *Population Studies* 33(2): 343–351.

Russett, Bruce and John Oneal. 2001. *Triangulating Peace: Democracy, Interdependence, and International Organizations.* New York: Norton.

Russett, Bruce M. 1969. "Who Pays for Defense?" *American Political Science Review* 63(2): 412–426.

Russett, Bruce M. 1970. "Comment on Defense Spending and Foreign Policy in the House of Representatives." *Journal of Conflict Resolution* 14(2): 287–290.

Russett, Bruce M. 1982. "Defense Expenditures and National Well-Being." *American Political Science Review* 76(4): 767–777.

Schmeidl, Susanne. 2000. "The Quest for Accuracy in the Estimation of Forced Migration." In Stephen C. Lubkemann, Larry Minear, and Thomas G. Weiss, eds., *Humanitarian Action: Social Science Connections*. Providence, RI: Thomas J. Watson Jr. Institute for International Studies, 127–157.

Sen, Amartya. 2000. "Why Human Security." Presentation at the International Symposium on Human Security, Tokyo, July 28.

Sen, Amartya. 2001. "Economic Progress and Health." In David Leon and Gill Walt, eds., *Poverty, Inequality, and Health*. Oxford: Oxford University Press, 333–345.

Shi, Michael E. 2002. "Income Inequality, Democracy, and Health: A Global Portrait." Paper presented at "Responding to Globalization: Societies, Groups, and Individuals," a conference held at the Institute of Behavioral Science, University of Colorado at Boulder, April 4–7.

Smith, R. P. 1977. "Military Expenditures and Capitalism." *Cambridge Journal of Economics* 1: 61–76.

Steiner, Henry and Philip Alston. 1996. *International Human Rights in Context: Law, Politics, and Morals*. Oxford: Oxford University Press.

Stewart, Frances and Valpy Fitzgerald. 2001. *War and Underdevelopment*, vol. 1: *The Economic and Social Consequences of Conflict*. Oxford: Oxford University Press.

Strand, Håvard, Joachim Carlsen, Nils Petter Gleditsch, Håvard Hegre, Christin Ormhaug, and Lars Wilhelmsen. 2005. *Armed Conflict Dataset Codebook, Version 3*. Oslo: International Peace Research Institute.

Taipale, Ilkka, ed. 2002. *War or Health? A Reader*. London: Zed Books.

Taubenberger, Jeffery. 1997. "Initial Genetic Characterization of the 1918 'Spanish' Influenza Virus." *Science* 275: 1793–1796.

Thakur, Ramesh. 1997. "From National to Human Security." In Stewart Harris and Andrew Mack, eds., *Asia-Pacific Security: The Economics-Politics Nexus*. Sydney: Allen and Unwin, 53–54.

Thompson, William. 1996. "Democracy and Peace: Putting the Cart Before the Horse?" *International Organization* 50(1): 141–174.

Tsui, Amy Ong. 2001. "Population Policies, Family Planning Programs, and Fertility: The Record." *Population and Development Review* 27(Supplement: Global Fertility Transition): 184–204.

Tsui, Amy Ong and Donald J. Bogue. 1978. "Declining World Fertility: Trends, Causes, and Implications." *Population Bulletin* 33(4): 1–55.

Ul Haq, Mahbub. 1999. "Global Governance for Human Security." In Maiid Tehranian, ed., *Worlds Apart: Human Security and Global Governance*. New York: I. B. Tauris, 73–94.

United Kingdom Department for International Development. 2003. "Bosnia: Health Briefing Paper." London: Health Systems Resource Center.

United Nations. 1946. *The Constitution of the World Health Organization.* New York: United Nations.

United Nations. 1948. *The Universal Declaration of Human Rights.* New York: United Nations.

United Nations Development Programme. 1994. *Human Development Report.* New York: United Nations Development Programme.

United Nations Development Programme. 2002. *Human Development Report.* New York: United Nations Development Programme.

United Nations Development Programme. 2003. *Human Development Report.* New York: United Nations Development Programme.

United Nations Development Programme. 2004. *Human Development Report.* New York: United Nations Development Programme.

United Nations High Commissioner for Refugees. 2005. *Helping Refugees: An Introduction to UNHCR.* Geneva: United Nations High Commissioner for Refugees.

United Nations High Commissioner for Refugees. 2006. *The State of the World's Refugees.* New York: Oxford University Press.

United Nations High Commissioner for Refugees. 2007. *Statistical Yearbook 2006: Trends in Displacement, Protection and Solutions.* Geneva: United Nations High Commissioner for Refugees.

Walter, Barbara. 1999. "Designing Transitions from Civil War: Demobilization, Democratization, and Commitments to Peace." *International Security* 24(1): 127–155.

Ward, Michael D. and David R. Davis. 1992. "Sizing up the Peace Dividend: Economic Growth and Military Spending in the United States, 1948–1996." *American Political Science Review* 86(3): 748–755.

Ward, Michael D., David R. Davis, and Corey L. Lofdahl. 1995. "A Century of Trade-Offs: Defense and Growth in Japan and the United States." *International Studies Quarterly* 39(1): 27–50.

Weiner, Myron. 1992. "Security, Stability, and International Migration." *International Security* 17(3): 91–126.

Weiner, Myron. 1996. "Bad Neighbors, Bad Neighborhoods: An Inquiry into the Causes of Refugee Flows." *International Security* 21(1): 5–42.

Weiss, Thomas G. 1999. "Whither International Efforts for Internally Displaced Persons?" *Journal of Peace Research* 36(3): 363–373.

Werner, Suzanne. 1998. "Negotiating the Terms of Settlement: War Aims and Bargaining Leverage." *Journal of Conflict Resolution* 42(3): 321–343.

Werner, Suzanne. 1999. "The Precarious Nature of Peace: Resolving the Issues, Enforcing the Settlement, and Renegotiating the Terms." *American Journal of Political Science* 43(3): 912–934.

Wilkinson, Richard G. 1996. *Unhealthy Societies: The Afflictions of Inequality.* London: Routledge.

World Bank. 2004. *World Development Indicators.* Washington, DC: World Bank Group.

World Bank. 2006. *World Development Index.* Washington, DC: World Bank Group.

World Health Organization. 1998a. *Health Conditions of the Population in Iraq Since the Gulf Crisis.* Geneva: World Health Organization.

World Health Organization. 1998b. *WHO's Humanitarian Activities in Iraq Under SCR 986.* Geneva: World Health Organization.

World Health Organization. 2000. *Global Situation in Reproductive and Family Health.* Geneva: World Health Organization.

World Health Organization. 2002a. *World Report on Violence and Health.* Geneva: World Health Organization.

World Health Organization. 2002b. *The World Health Report 2002.* Geneva: World Health Organization.

World Health Organization. 2003. *Liberia Health Update: 5 September 2003.* Geneva: World Health Organization.

Zellner, Arnold. 1962. "An Efficient Method of Estimating Seemingly Unrelated Regressions and Tests for Aggregation Bias." *Journal of the American Statistical Association* 57(298): 348–368.

Zorn, Christopher. 2001. "Generalized Estimating Equation Models for Correlated Data: A Review with Applications." *American Journal of Political Science* 45(2): 470–490.

Zwi, Anthony. 2001. "Injuries, Inequalities, and Health: From Policy Vacuum to Policy Action." In David Leon and Gill Walt, eds., *Poverty, Inequality, and Health.* Oxford: Oxford University Press, 263–282.

INDEX